Practical
Insulin Therapy

Practical Insulin Therapy

Pradeep G Talwalkar MD FICA FICP
Senior Consultant Diabetologist
SL Raheja Hospital
All India Institute of Diabetes, Mumbai
Formerly Honorary Professor of Medicine
Grant Medical College
Mumbai, Maharashtra, India

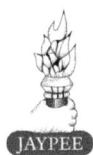

JAYPEE BROTHERS MEDICAL PUBLISHERS
The Health Sciences Publisher
New Delhi | London

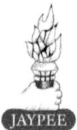 **Jaypee Brothers Medical Publishers (P) Ltd**

Headquarters
EMCA House
23/23-B, Ansari Road, Daryaganj
New Delhi 110 002, India
Landline: +91-11-23272143, +91-11-23272703
+91-11-23282021, +91-11-23245672
E-mail: jaypee@jaypeebrothers.com

Corporate Office
Jaypee Brothers Medical Publishers (P) Ltd.
4838/24, Ansari Road, Daryaganj
New Delhi 110 002, India
Phone: +91-11-43574357
Fax: +91-11-43574314
E-mail: jaypee@jaypeebrothers.com

Overseas Office
JP Medical Ltd.
83, Victoria Street, London
SW1H 0HW (UK)
Phone: +44-20 3170 8910
E-mail: info@jpmedpub.com

EU GPSR Authorised Representative
Logos Europe, 9 rue Nicolas Poussin
17000, La Rochelle, France
Phone: +33 (0) 6 67 93 73 78
E-mail: Contact@logoseurope.eu

Website: www.jaypeebrothers.com
Website: www.jaypeedigital.com

© 2024, Jaypee Brothers Medical Publishers

The views and opinions expressed in this book are solely those of the original contributor(s)/author(s) and do not necessarily represent those of editor(s) or publisher of the book.

All rights reserved. No part of this publication may be reproduced, stored or transmitted in any form or by any means, electronic, mechanical, photocopying, recording or otherwise, without the prior permission in writing of the publishers.

All brand names and product names used in this book are trade names, service marks, trademarks or registered trademarks of their respective owners. The publisher is not associated with any product or vendor mentioned in this book.

Medical knowledge and practice change constantly. This book is designed to provide accurate, authoritative information about the subject matter in question. However, readers are advised to check the most current information available on procedures included and check information from the manufacturer of each product to be administered, to verify the recommended dose, formula, method and duration of administration, adverse effects and contraindications. It is the responsibility of the practitioner to take all appropriate safety precautions. Neither the publisher nor the author(s)/editor(s) assume any liability for any injury and/or damage to persons or property arising from or related to use of material in this book.

This book is sold on the understanding that the publisher is not engaged in providing professional medical services. If such advice or services are required, the services of a competent medical professional should be sought.

Every effort has been made where necessary to contact holders of copyright to obtain permission to reproduce copyright material. If any have been inadvertently overlooked, the publisher will be pleased to make the necessary arrangements at the first opportunity.

Inquiries for bulk sales may be solicited at: jaypee@jaypeebrothers.com

Practical Insulin Therapy / Pradeep G Talwalkar

First Edition: **2024**

ISBN: 978-93-5696-538-6

Dedicated to

My late parents
Dr Gopal Vasudeo Talvalkar (MD)
and
Mrs Indumati Gopal Talwalkar (MA English Literature)

Preface

Today, India is in the midst of an exciting and challenging period. The epidemic of diabetes in India is still intensifying by leaps and bounds and we already have 101 million people with diabetes. The rapid improvement in the socio-economic status of our people has further accelerated, along with remarkable improvement in the availability of medical facilities and the affordability of people to avail them. Rapid urbanization, westernization, and industrialization have contributed to a further increase in the prevalence of diabetes, and at the same time, the longevity of our population has remarkably increased. Thus, people with diabetes live longer and a higher percentage of them are reaching the stage of β-cell failure, thus requiring insulin for glycemic control.

Majority of people with diabetes are treated by primary and secondary care physicians who have high workload. They require a concise but at the same time comprehensive source of "predigested", ready-to-use contemporary and reliable information, which they would like to keep on their clinic table for regular reference. Thus, I am making this sincere attempt to address the needs of practitioners of our country through the First Edition of *Practical Insulin Therapy*.

Pradeep G Talwalkar

Acknowledgments

I thank innumerable primary and secondary care physicians who have expressed their appreciation of my style of medical writing and thus encouraged me to keep on writing for them. My thanks are due to my wife, Dr Vandana, whose support, encouragement, help, and sacrifice led to the successful culmination of my efforts. My thanks are also due to Dr Saumya Chatterjee, Mrs Ashwini Kunte, Mr Jitendra Kamble, and many other well-wishers in industry, who provided inputs such as compilation of data on availability of insulin preparations in the Indian market and illustrations on insulin regimens.

I thank Shri Jitendar P Vij (Group Chairman), Mr Ankit Vij (Managing Director), Mr MS Mani (Group President), Ms Chetna Malhotra (Senior Director—Professional Publishing, Marketing, and Business Development), Ms Pooja Bhandari [Director—Production (Books and Journals)], Mrs Kritika Dua (Commissioning Editor), and Mr Priyansh Saxena (Development Editor), M/s Jaypee Brothers Medical Publishers (P) Ltd, New Delhi, India, for constant encouragement.

Pradeep G Talwalkar

Contents

1. Introduction — 1
2. Discovery of Insulin — 4
3. Evolution of Insulin Therapy — 9
4. Insulin Physiology and Pathophysiology in Diabetes Mellitus — 19
5. Biosimilar Insulin — 25
6. Insulin Resistance — 29
7. Insulin in the Management of Diabetes — 36
8. Hypoglycemia with Insulin Therapy — 74
9. Insulin Delivery Systems — 81
10. Insulin Preparations Available in India — 104

Index — 115

CHAPTER 1

Introduction

Diabetes mellitus is principally a disease of insulin deficiency, either absolute as in type 1 diabetes mellitus (T1DM), or relative, as in type 2 diabetes mellitus (T2DM). Without insulin deficiency, diabetes cannot develop. Varying degree of insulin resistance is usually associated with insulin deficiency in T2DM and acquired faulty lifestyle-related insulin resistance can develop in those with T1DM, but insulin resistance is not a prerequisite for its development. Insulin is an important anabolic hormone closely involved in carbohydrate, fat, and protein metabolism. The principal action of insulin is to control blood glucose level and keep it in a normal range by facilitating its entry into tissues such as skeletal muscles and fat where it is partly metabolized to release energy and partly stored as glycogen for future use. Insulin also suppresses hepatic glucose production. Injected insulin directly tackles insulin deficiency and thus, it works in all types of diabetes and at all stages. It has no contraindication. All noninsulin antidiabetic agents have some contraindications and limitations.

Insulin is secreted by β-cells, which along with other endocrine cells such as α-cells are present in small clusters or islands called islets of Langerhans spread across the pancreas. β-cells make up about 1–2% of pancreatic mass. Insulin deficiency leads to diabetes mellitus. Management of diabetes involves correction of hyperglycemia with appropriate medical nutritional therapy, exercise, and antidiabetic medications. Simultaneous swift and persistent control of associated abnormalities such as elevated blood pressure and deranged levels of lipids is equally important. Patients with T1DM have total insulin deficiency and under such circumstances externally administered insulin is the only available therapeutic agent in the management of hyperglycemia. Thus, once T1DM fully sets in, life beyond a few weeks is not possible without insulin administration. Hence, till the introduction of insulin into clinical practice, diagnosis of T1DM was considered as an unofficial death sentence. T2DM is a disease characterized by progressive reduction in β-cell function associated with progressively reducing insulin secretion and release in circulation. Though several noninsulin agents having different mechanisms of action, often complimentary to each other, are available for management of hyperglycemia in patients with T2DM, they all have limited capacities to reduce glycated hemoglobin (HbA1c). Furthermore, among all the groups with moderate to strong capacity to reduce HbA1c, sodium-glucose cotransporter-2 (SGLT-2) inhibitors are the only agents which work in the absence of insulin in an environment. In such situations, other noninsulin antidiabetic agents are totally or significantly ineffective. Thus, majority of long-standing T2DM patients require insulin in addition to these agents or to replace them.

■ CASE STUDY

Mr SK, aged 66 years, has been a known diabetic patient for 12 years. Currently, he is on 2 g of metformin, 6 mg of glimepiride and 100 mg of sitagliptin daily. His HbA1c is 10.2% and estimated glomerular filtration rate (eGFR) is 35 mL/min/1.73 m². SK and his doctor agree that he needs better glycemic control. What are their choices or is there any choice other than insulin? Let us discuss.

Since SK's eGFR is lower than 45 mL/min/1.73 m², he requires to reduce his metformin dosage by 50%, glimepiride is already in high dose, any further increase is unlikely to give any significant improvement in glycemic control. Sitagliptin is already in full therapeutic dosage but actually its dosage should be reduced by 50% in view of moderately severe renal insufficiency. Long-standing status of diabetes coupled with very high HbA1c in spite of three agents with different and synergistic antidiabetic actions indicates advanced β-cell failure and severe insulin deficiency. Reduction of metformin dose by 50%, which is essential, is very likely to worsen glycemic control significantly.

Let us consider available agents:
- *SGLT-2 inhibitors*: The average capacity to reduce HbA1c is 0.8–0.9%, furthermore as eGFR decreases, their glycemic efficacy reduces progressively. Thus, in SK's case they will mainly work as renoprotective agents and are not expected to make significant contribution toward reducing HbA1c and bringing it to the goal.
- *Glucagon-like peptide-1 receptor agonists (GLP-1 RAs)*: These are a bit more efficacious as compared to SGLT-2 inhibitors and their glycemic efficacy is retained in renal impairment; however, significant percentage of their antidiabetic action is dependent on viability of β-cells. Furthermore, when GLP-1 RA comes on board, sitagliptin is superfluous and will have to be removed. Thus, net overall effect on HbA1c will be smaller. Furthermore, high cost of these agents, (around ₹9,000/- month), is a major limiting factor in our country where a majority of patients spend on their medications out of pocket.
- *Pioglitazone*: It has the capacity to reduce HbA1c by about 1% and renal impairment is theoretically not a contraindication for its use. However, long-standing T2DM patients with chronic renal impairment are very likely to have cardiovascular disease even if it is not clinically obvious and

thus SK will need through cardiac evaluation to rule out cardiac failure, which is a contraindication for its use. Side effects such as edema and weight gain can come up, leading to the need for withdrawal or use in smaller dosages such as 7.5 mg/day. Pioglitazone requires presence of insulin to produce its glycemic action, either natural insulin from β-cells, or externally administered. SK appears to be near end stage β-cell failure and thus pioglitazone is unlikely to be fully effective.

- *Alpha-glucosidase inhibitors*: These agents have ability to reduce HbA1c by about 0.5%, predominantly working on postprandial glycemic excursions. They are contraindicated in those with moderate or higher stages of renal impairment.

Thus, even if SK's HbA1c target is fixed at 7.2–7.5% and even if all the four classes of agents are brought on board, he will not be able to reach the target or stay at it in a durable manner.

From the discussion above, a reader will clearly understand that even if SK had HbA1c of 9.7%, and eGFR of 50, he would not be able to reach his glycemic goal or stay at it durably unless insulin is brought on board.

India has 101 million people with diabetes, >95% of these are T2DM patients. The prevalence of diabetes is increasing by leaps and bounds. Diabetics are living longer and thus the number of insulin requiring patients with T2DM is also steeply increasing. However, due to severe insulin phobia and inertia to start insulin, a large number of patients go shopping from doctor to doctor in search of someone who will prescribe some magic pill and bring his HbA1c to the set goal. On average, Indian patients start insulin about 8 years after it is due and when their HbA1c is well beyond 9.0%. The main reason for higher prevalence of microvascular, macrovascular; and infectious diseases complications of diabetes in Indian patients is comparatively poorer glycemic control due to very late acceptance of insulin therapy.

The majority of these patients are being treated by generalists, general physicians, and family physicians with varying experience, expertise, and knowledge about the disease and its management. Practical insulin therapy is a concise book which covers all the information needed by the practitioner to confidently start insulin in appropriate patients. The confidence he will get after reading the book will go a long way in shedding inertia, (if at all he has it) and positively convincing the patient to accept insulin therapy without delaying the decision to start it and reaping the benefits that will be derived from better glycemic control.

CHAPTER 2

Discovery of Insulin

■ INTRODUCTION

The discovery of insulin and its introduction in clinical practice were major milestones not only in the field of diabetes management but in the larger field of medical science and therapeutics. Before the advent of insulin, diagnosis of type 1 diabetes mellitus (T1DM) meant a death sentence. Now, 100 years later, many people with T1DM are living a long, high-quality, productive life. The journey of discovery of insulin and the subsequent ongoing, gradual, progressive improvement in purity, quality, and capabilities of newer insulin, from bovine to porcine to human to analog insulin, along with impressive improvements in devices to administer insulin, is a fascinating story. Though the credit of discovery rightfully goes to Banting, Best, and Macleod, decades of hard work by several doctors and scientists from different disciplines working in laboratories and clinics across north America and Europe was also very crucial. These scientists, often working individually and oblivious of what others are doing and achieving in the same areas of research, had generated a significant base of knowledge, which worked as a springboard for Banting to visualize, conceptualize, and give directions to his project of discovering a natural substance, later nomenclated as insulin, which could dramatically make a positive change in lives of patients having diabetes. Thus, it is worth reviewing important milestones in relevant research in the preinsulin era.

■ IMPORTANT RESEARCH MILESTONES IN THE PREINSULIN ERA

Pancreas was first described by Greek anatomist and surgeon Herophilus (335–280 BC). Swiss anatomist and surgeon, JC Brunner first performed pancreatectomy in 1663, however there was no further progress in understanding details of structure and function of pancreas for two more centuries. In 1869, Paul Langerhans, a medical student in Berlin, was the first to identify clumps of cells scattered throughout the body of pancreas. These clumps were later named islets of Langerhans. Edouard Laguesse suggested that the secretions from these cells could have a role in digestion. In 1889, Oscar Minkowski, in collaboration with Joseph Mering, removed the pancreas from a healthy dog to verify its role in digestion. Observations which surprised both the scientists included excessive urination and several flies getting attracted toward dog's urine which was everywhere in the doghouse. In addition, the finding of glucose in pancreatectomized dog's urine gave a strong clue for future scientists working on finding treatments for diabetes, who then concentrated on making extracts from islets and verifying their effects on pancreatectomized dogs. In 1901, an American physician, Eugene Lindsay Opie stated, *"diabetes is caused by lesions of islets of Langerhans, either complete destruction, or part destruction".* In 1906, George Ludwig Zuelzer achieved partial success in pancreatectomized dog with pancreatic extract but left the project halfway. In 1911, EL Scott at the University of Chicago tried aqueous pancreatic extract and got partial success, however, further work was not pursued due to lack of support from superiors. In 1916, Nicolae Paulescu achieved good success with pancreatic extract, but due to the eruption of the First World War, his project was stalled.

■ DISCOVERY OF INSULIN

At the beginning of the 1920s, it was clear that extract from islets of Langerhans had therapeutic properties against diabetes and it was needed in concentrated form to have meaningful beneficial effects. It was also known that pancreatic enzymes could destroy islet cell secretion.

Enter Frederick Banting, a young surgeon in London, Ontario, Canada, struggling to establish his practice. In order to earn some fixed income on the side, he took a part-time demonstrator's job at a local medical school. One night, while preparing for the next day's lecture on pancreas, he came across an article titled "relation of islets of Langerhans to diabetes, with special reference to cases of pancreatic lithiasis". In this article, Barron from the University of Minnesota had described the autopsy findings that included degeneration of acinar cells due to total blockade of main pancreatic duct by calculus, with relative preservation of islets of Langerhans. His sharp mind immediately developed *"eureka"* feeling (*"I have found it"*), he developed an idea to ligate pancreatic duct of dogs and to keep them alive till acini degenerate and then sacrifice the dog, remove pancreas and extract concentrated form of islets secretions and to subsequently try them on pancreatectomized dogs. In order to acquire funding, research infrastructure and an assistant to help him in his research work, he approached Professor Robert Macleod, Professor of Physiology at the University of Toronto and a leading authority in physiology. The professor was initially not convinced about the feasibility of Banting's proposed project but, after repeated pleas, the professor appreciated Banting's conviction, resolve and total involvement, accepted the project and provided for the financial and logistic requirements. When the post for assistant research worker was advertised, there were two eager and eligible applicants. Thus, it was split and the coin was tossed to decide who would work in the first half of the project. The coin toss favored Charles Best, a medical student, in pursuit of gainfully utilizing his vacation period and he was selected to assist Banting in the first half of the project period. He was given special training to estimate blood glucose levels, which was required to assess the efficacy of their pancreatic extract.

On 17th May 1921, a team of three, Banting, main proponent and lead investigator, but a surgeon by training, Best, the medical student who volunteered to be a research assistant and was given specific responsibility of blood glucose measurement, and Professor Macleod who assumed the role of advisor, was formed. They started work on tying pancreatic duct, wait for acinar degeneration, followed by sacrificing the dog and extracting pancreatic material and then injecting it in pancreatectomized dog and studying its effects on blood and urine glucose levels and clinical status of the dog. The success was slow. Besides setbacks on the scientific front, there were major setbacks on the logistic front. Macleod took a long time to get convinced about the future of the project and, thus, funding for provisions as well as Banting's salary was threatened. Personal relations between Best and Macleod were at a nadir. However, the team persisted and perseverance ultimately paid off.

By *November 1921*, they had successfully treated a pancreatectomized dog named Marjorie, with resultant diabetes with their insulin extract for 70 days. In their noting on the experiments, Banting and Best labeled the pancreatic extract as isletin. At this stage, Banting decided to purify pancreatic extract for better results as well as to make the extract suitable for injections in humans. Banting asked for the help of James Collip, an expert biochemist with a special interest and aptitude in protein purification. Collip was on the way back to his hometown after returning from a study tour of the USA and was doing his sabbatical at the department of pathological chemistry at the University of Toronto. After initially refusing to take Collip on board, Macleod relented. Collip worked day and night on purification of pancreatic extract.

On 11th January 1922, human grade purified pancreatic extract was injected into master Leonard Thompson, a 14-year-old dying patient with T1DM, in Toronto General Hospital, Canada. Leonard survived and his blood glucose dropped considerably, but ketosis could not be reversed and he developed abscess at injection site, indicating clear need for further purification of pancreatic extract. Collip worked hard and further purified pancreatic extract and purified extract was injected in to Master Leonard Thompson on 23rd January 1922. This time there was a reduction in blood glucose level to near normal associated with significant clinical improvement and no obvious side effects. Thus, Leonard's death sentence was *"reversed"*.

On 3rd May 1922, Macleod announced the discovery of insulin to international medical community at the meeting of Association of American Physicians. He read a paper titled "The Effects Produced on Diabetes by Extracts of Pancreas". He used the word "insulin" for the first time.

On 23rd January 1923, US patent on insulin and its method of manufacturing was awarded to Banting, Collip, and Best. They all sold the patent to the University of Toronto for a nominal sum of $1. Banting who was a selfless researcher and a gentleman, made a statement, *"insulin does not belong to me, it belongs to everyone".* He wanted everybody who needed insulin to have easy access to it.

On 15th October 1923, as the success of insulin therapy in diabetics spread, the demand increased by leaps and bounds, researchers started work on scaling up production of insulin. Eli Lilly became the first commercial company to start producing insulin on a large scale.

On 25th October 1923, in recognition of their lifesaving discovery of insulin, Banting and Macleod were jointly awarded the 1923 Nobel Prize in physiology or medicine. Banting shared his prize with Best, while Macleod shared his prize with Collip.

Thus, the long-drawn-out saga of insulin discovery ended with a big victory for Banting, the main hero or the central figure in the story. The story of discovery of insulin has many similarities with a typical multi-starrer masala Bollywood movie. Multiple characters, several ups and downs, coincidences, serendipity; and ultimately, a big victory for good or deserving over bad or nondeserving, are the similarities. However, the main difference is, while the discovery of insulin was a revolutionary event with far-reaching benefits for millions of patients with diabetes all over the globe, masala Bollywood movie is good enough only to pass time for couple of hours.

■ SUMMARY

The discovery of insulin revolutionized the management of diabetes, particularly T1DM. It is a fascinating story involving several scientists in different geographies of the western hemisphere, often working independently and oblivious of outcomes of research work being done by other research workers. The process leading to the discovery was a long drawn out and faced several scientific and logistic roadblocks on the way. Ultimately, the hard work, perseverance and self-belief displayed by Dr Banting and his group succeeded and the discovery of insulin revolutionized the management of diabetes.

CHAPTER 2: Discovery of Insulin

■ BANTING AND HIS TEAM WHO DISCOVERED INSULIN

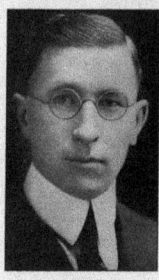
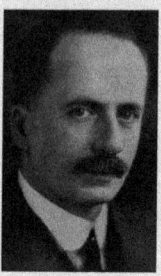
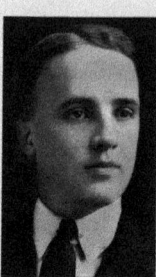
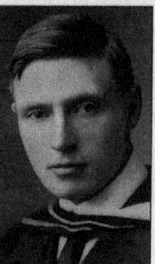

Frederick Grant Banting 1891–1941   John James Rickard Macleod 1876–1935   Charles Crochet Best 1899–1978   James Bertram Collip 1892–1965

1. *Dr Frederick Grant Banting (1891-1941)*: The leader of the team, who conceptualized and drove the research project on discovery of insulin. Surgeon by qualification, who later became a full-time researcher.
2. *Professor John James Rickard Macleod (1876-1935)*: Professor of Physiology at the University of Toronto. He provided general guidance to research project of Dr Banting and also provided logistic support to Dr Banting in his department at University of Toronto. He jointly received a Nobel prize in 1923 along with Dr Banting for the discovery of insulin.
3. *Dr Charles Best (1899-1978)*: Dr Best was a medical student and joined Dr Banting as a research assistant in the summer vacation of 1921. He received training on estimation of blood glucose and worked hard on the entire project, side by side with Dr Banting, who shared his Nobel prize money with Dr Best.
4. *Professor James Bertram Collip (1892-1965)*: Professor Collip was a biochemist with a special interest in protein purification. When the need to further purify the pancreatic extract made by Dr Banting was acutely felt, Dr Banting requested Professor Macleod to induct Professor Collip in his research team. His knowledge about purification of proteins and hard work in the insulin project played a key role in the ultimate success of the project. In the recognition of his contribution, Dr Macleod shared the Nobel prize money with Professor James Collip.

CHAPTER 3

Evolution of Insulin Therapy

■ INTRODUCTION

"Insulin" which Master Leonard Thompson received on January 19, 1921 was a murky light brown liquid with significant sedimentation and had to be heated before subcutaneous injection to increase its solubility. It was 1:1 mixture of beef pancreas extract and alcohol. In the case papers at Toronto General Hospital, in Canada, where it was administered to a human being for the first time ever, it was mentioned as "Dr McLeod's serum." It was officially christened a few months later as insulin. There was a significant drop in blood glucose after the first injection but ketosis persisted and Master Thompson developed an injection site abscess. Obviously, it was too impure to continue. Collip, the fourth member of the team that discovered insulin, and a biochemist with a special interest in protein purification, who was working day and night on the purification of pancreatic extract and improving its purity continuously as an ongoing process even before it was administered to master Thompson on January 19, 1921 increased alcohol content of extract and improved it further. Master Thompson received his second dose of insulin on January 23, 2023. This time, the improvement in blood glucose was far greater and there were no side effects. Since then, there has been continuous ongoing improvement in evolutionary manner as regards purification, structure, pharmacokinetic capabilities, suitability for individual needs, reduction in side effects, modes of administration, etc. Insulin analogs which we use today in day-to-day clinical practice with precise administration devices are poles apart from murky light brown precipitate which was injected in Master Thompson's subcutaneous tissue with a crude metallic syringe and a blunt needle resulting in unbearable pain, 100 years ago. Let us review this fascinating, ever-evolving journey of 100 years.

■ PURITY OF INSULIN

Though the second dose of insulin received by Master Thompson was better, it still had many impurities which included several other proteins from pancreatic extract. Purification of insulin was a continuous process till the introduction of genetically engineered human insulin in the market.

In the initial experiments, dog pancreatic extract was used. Subsequently, bovine pancreatic extract was the starting material for purification. In 1923, Illy Lilley was the first company to mass-market insulin for the first time under the Iletin brand. In 1926, the first progress toward insulin purification occurred through the availability of insulin crystals. The conventional bovine insulin was purified by the process involving a series of isoelectric precipitations and recrystallizations. However, in spite of the method of purification, conventional insulin contained some impurities in the form of proinsulin, glucagon, pancreatic poly peptides, somatostatin, vasoactive intestinal polypeptides, etc., in very small amounts.

In the seventies, highly purified bovine insulin, soon followed by monocomponent bovine insulin was introduced. Improved purity led to reduced chances of significant anti-insulin antibodies and reduced chances of therapy-related insulin resistance.

STRUCTURE OF INSULIN

The structural difference between bovine, porcine, and human insulin is enumerated in **Table 1**.

The insulin molecule consists of two polypeptide chains. The shorter "A" chain contains 21 amino acids while the longer "B" chain contains 30 amino acids. Bovine insulin differs from human insulin by three amino acids (two in the "A" chain at the 8 and 10th positions and one in the "B" chain at the 30th position). Porcine and human insulin have an identical "A" chain while it differs by only one amino acid (at 30th position in the "B" chain). The following table shows species of insulin and the corresponding amino acids at the 8th and 10th positions in the "A" chain and the 30th position in the "B" chain (at all other positions in both chains, the amino acids are identical) **(Table 1)**.

The aforementioned structural differences between bovine and porcine insulin with human insulin were responsible for systemic allergic reactions that were occasionally seen in clinical practice. Since porcine insulin differs from human insulin by only one amino acid, the prevalence of allergy to porcine insulin is less than that to bovine insulin.

TABLE 1: Structural differences between bovine, porcine, and human insulin.			
	"A" chain		"B" chain
Type of insulin	8th position	10th position	30th position
Bovine	Alanine	Valine	Alanine
Porcine	Threonine	Isoleucine	Alanine
Human	Threonine	Isoleucine	Threonine

The commercially available human insulin is immunologically identical to insulin produced in the human islets of Langerhans, hence allergic reactions to human insulin are extremely rare and are obviously due to the presence of additives and preservatives.

Besides the above-mentioned differences, human insulin has a neutral pH while conventional animal crystalline insulin has an acidic pH. Neutral pH makes them more stable and more compatible with the tissues.

Besides problems related to structural differences, demand–supply mismatch of raw material (bovine/porcine pancreas) was a major bottleneck leading to inadequate supply of finished insulin in the market. This also led to cost escalation. In advanced countries, porcine insulin was introduced soon after bovine insulin, while it was introduced in the Indian market around 1980 and it was costlier than bovine insulin. Thus, though it reduced immunological issues to some extent, availability problems persisted. All these issues were automatically eliminated when human insulin was introduced in the market. Human insulin was initially manufactured by a semisynthetic process for a short period. The manufacturing was subsequently upgraded to biosynthetic method using genetic engineering technology, [recombinant deoxyribonucleic acid (DNA) technology]. In this process, a plasmid is isolated from a bacterium (*Escherichia coli*) or a fungus (*Saccharomyces*) and cut open. Insulin-producing gene from β-cells in the pancreas is then inserted in the plasmid and both are recombined together by DNA ligase enzyme and inserted into suitable host (*E. coli* or *Saccharomyces*) which starts synthesizing insulin. A chain and B chain are produced separately by an identical process and then both the chains are joined together to form the complete insulin molecule having 51 amino acids. Thus, the introduction of genetically engineered human insulin, which has exactly the same structure as that of native human insulin secreted by β-cells in the pancreas, has eliminated several issues, such as immunogenicity, raw material shortage, lipodystrophy at the injection site, and availability at one go and has made animal insulin redundant. This was a major milestone in the continuous evolution of insulin development. Human insulin was commercially introduced in 1982.

LONGER-ACTING INSULIN

Insulin introduced in clinical practice initially was a short-acting insulin and thus, besides its purity problems, major additional drawbacks were the need for multiple daily injections to cover all major meals and the inability to maintain adequate hepatic insulinization throughout the night without producing hypoglycemia. Soon after the introduction of insulin in clinical practice, work on the development of longer-acting insulin was started. Different proteins such as protamine and globulin were combined with insulin in a suspension to prolong its duration of action. The developmental work in this direction ultimately led to the introduction of isophane insulin in 1946 on the market. The addition of a protein (protamine), along with zinc and phenol in suspension form leads to slower absorption from the subcutaneous tissue and thus prolongation of duration of action. After subcutaneous injection, it starts acting in 90 minutes, has a peak of around 6–10 hours and duration of action of 10–16 hours. Since its action is not long enough to maintain therapeutically effective blood levels for 24 hours; it is classified as intermediate-acting insulin. In 1952, lente insulin with a similar pharmacokinetic profile was introduced in clinical practice and withdrawn subsequently as it could not match the stability of neutral protamine Hagedorn (NPH) insulin.

■ PREMIXED INSULIN

After the introduction of NPH insulin, thrice-a-day short-acting insulin along with once or twice-a-day NPH insulin became the gold standard basal-bolus therapy in all type 1 diabetes mellitus (T1DM) and many type 2 diabetes mellitus (T2DM) patients with poor β-cell reserve or with complications driven by severe insulin resistance. Some patients, particularly elderly patients, were not comfortable with self-mixing of short-acting and intermediate-acting insulin and, at the same time, not ready to accept multiple injections daily. The development and introduction of fixed-dose, premixed combinations of short- and intermediate-acting insulin was the industry's response. At present 30:70 and 50:50 combinations (short-acting:intermediate-acting) are freely available. Premixed insulin provides convenience at the cost of precision. In the hands of a learned and experienced clinician, it is a pragmatic option in carefully selected patients. More information on the pros and cons of premixed insulin is given in the appropriate chapter.

■ INHALED INSULIN

Inhaled ultrashort-acting human insulin was developed for prandial blood glucose control especially for those T1DM and T2DM patients who are averse to taking multiple insulin injections, they can combine inhaled insulin at each meal with one injection of long-acting insulin, and T2DM patients with predominant postprandial hyperglycemia in spite of taking multiple OADs and desiring to improve glycemic control without restoring to insulin injections. Use of a large pulmonary alveolar surface is gainfully utilized for rapid absorption of powdered human insulin packaged in a cartridge and inhaled through a small inhaler. Launched in the USA in 2015, it serves the needs of patients who are hell-bent on avoiding insulin or avoiding more than one injection per 24 hours. Its pharmacokinetic profile is similar to that of ultrarapid-acting injectable insulin.

■ INSULIN ANALOGS

After genetically engineered human insulin, the introduction of insulin analogs was a major milestone in the evolution of insulin. Insulin analogs are altered forms of human insulin. Through genetic engineering of the underlying DNA, the amino acid sequence of insulin can be changed to suitably alter the absorption, distribution, metabolism, and excretion characteristics of human insulin without reducing their glycemic efficacy and also ensuring that their mitogenicity is not increased. In rapid-acting analogs, the altered structure is responsible for their faster absorption in circulation and quicker elimination. The first pharmacokinetic alteration can lead to better postprandial blood glucose control, while the later pharmacokinetic alteration can lead to lesser chances of late postprandial hypoglycemia. Precise alteration in amino acid structure, the resultant change in pharmacokinetic profile, and its clinical advantages over human insulin are discussed in Chapter 7. Lispro was the first insulin analog to be introduced in clinical practice by Eli Lilly Company in 1996 and was followed by Novo Nordisk's aspart insulin (1998). Both are examples of rapid-acting insulin. Sanofi's glulisine is the third rapid-acting insulin analog.

Just as there was a need for rapidly acting insulin for better postprandial glycemic control and lesser postprandial hypoglycemia, there was an even greater need for a long-acting insulin providing therapeutic plasma insulin levels for 24 hours and thus effectively providing basal insulin to suppress nighttime hepatic glucose production and at the same time reducing episodes of hypoglycemia, particularly severe and nocturnal hypoglycemia. Scientists working in research and development departments of major insulin-producing European countries successfully developed long-acting and ultra-long-acting insulin analogs and introduced glargine (2000), detemir (2005), degludec (2013), and glargine 300 (2015) in clinical practice. The desired pharmacokinetics were achieved by working on the amino acid sequence as well as by adding side chains to the amino acid structure for longer combination with subcutaneous tissue, and additionally as in the case of glargine, by changing the pH of insulin preparation.

Another major development or step forward in insulin therapy was the introduction of a coformulation of a rapid-acting insulin analog, aspart, with ultra-long-acting analog, degludec in the 30/70 format in 2013. Earlier premixed combinations with rapid-acting analogs were available (aspart with NPH and lispro with NPH). These formulations overcame the drawbacks of short-acting insulin but their longer-acting counterpart did not have 24-hour action; hence, these formulations were not suitable for once-a-day therapy in the majority and were associated with a higher prevalence of hypoglycemia, coformulation of aspart with degludec has very effectively overcome this drawback. Another advantage of this coformulation is that both the components are in solution and retain their individual identity on electrophoresis and also their individual pharmacokinetic properties. Furthermore, there is no need for shaking the formulation before each injection as it is not in suspension form.

Subsequent to the availability of long-acting and ultra-long-acting insulin analogs, ultrarapid-acting versions of aspart (Fiasp) (2018) and lispro (ultrarapid lispro) (2020) were introduced. These analogs get absorbed even quicker as compared to rapid-acting insulin analogs and offer better control of 1-hour postprandial blood glucose levels. In Fiasp niacinamide is added to aspart for further increase in speed of absorption, while in ultrarapid-acting lispro, treprostinil and citrate are added as expedients to facilitate faster absorption. Ultrarapid-acting insulin analog is a small step forward over rapid-acting insulin analogs in the ever-evolving insulin therapy scenario. All the aforementioned insulin analogs except ultrarapid-acting lispro are easily available in India.

■ CONCENTRATED INSULIN

Another direction in which insulin has evolved over the years is the development of concentrated insulin. In patients with severe insulin resistance, injection of large doses of insulin is associated with some disadvantages, such as large volume of injections, which can cause pain or discomfort, and the need for frequent refill prescriptions for insulin vials or pens, which can cause logistic problems. Following insulin products were developed to take care of these problems: (1) U-500 and U-200 short-acting insulin, (2) U-200 degludec, and (3) U-200 lispro. Out of these, U-200 short-acting insulin and U-200 lispro insulin are available in India. All the aforementioned variants have the same pharmacokinetics as those of corresponding U-100 insulin. Formulations with higher concentrations with special manufacturing technology to alter the pharmacokinetics are also available **(Fig. 1)** (glargine 300). In this example, the main purpose of development was to prolong the duration of action.

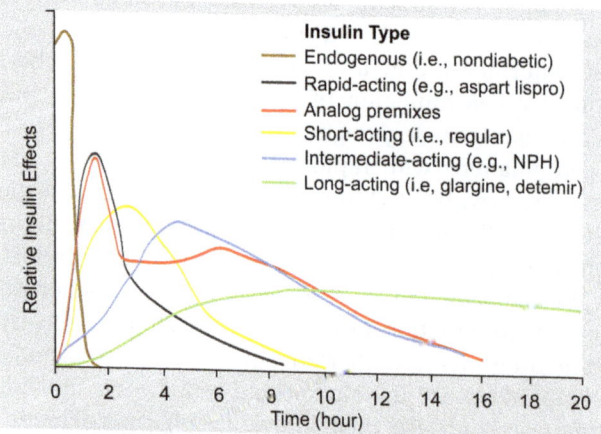

FIG. 1: Pharmacokinetic profiles of human insulin and insulin analogs.

Source: Freeman JS. Insulin analog therapy: improving the match with physiologic insulin secretion. J Am Osteopath Assoc. 2009;109(1):26-36. Quoted by White JR Insulin analogs: what are the clinical implications of structural differences? US Pharm. 2010;35(5)(Diabetes Suppl):3-7.

altered forms of human insulin. Through genetic engineering of the underlying DNA, the amino acid sequence of insulin can be changed to suitably alter the absorption, distribution, metabolism, and excretion characteristics of human insulin without reducing their glycemic efficacy and also ensuring that their mitogenicity is not increased. In rapid-acting analogs, the altered structure is responsible for their faster absorption in circulation and quicker elimination. The first pharmacokinetic alteration can lead to better postprandial blood glucose control, while the later pharmacokinetic alteration can lead to lesser chances of late postprandial hypoglycemia. Precise alteration in amino acid structure, the resultant change in pharmacokinetic profile, and its clinical advantages over human insulin are discussed in Chapter 7. Lispro was the first insulin analog to be introduced in clinical practice by Eli Lilly Company in 1996 and was followed by Novo Nordisk's aspart insulin (1998). Both are examples of rapid-acting insulin. Sanofi's glulisine is the third rapid-acting insulin analog.

Just as there was a need for rapidly acting insulin for better postprandial glycemic control and lesser postprandial hypoglycemia, there was an even greater need for a long-acting insulin providing therapeutic plasma insulin levels for 24 hours and thus effectively providing basal insulin to suppress nighttime hepatic glucose production and at the same time reducing episodes of hypoglycemia, particularly severe and nocturnal hypoglycemia. Scientists working in research and development departments of major insulin-producing European countries successfully developed long-acting and ultra-long-acting insulin analogs and introduced glargine (2000), detemir (2005), degludec (2013), and glargine 300 (2015) in clinical practice. The desired pharmacokinetics were achieved by working on the amino acid sequence as well as by adding side chains to the amino acid structure for longer combination with subcutaneous tissue, and additionally as in the case of glargine, by changing the pH of insulin preparation.

Another major development or step forward in insulin therapy was the introduction of a coformulation of a rapid-acting insulin analog, aspart, with ultra-long-acting analog, degludec in the 30/70 format in 2013. Earlier premixed combinations with rapid-acting analogs were available (aspart with NPH and lispro with NPH). These formulations overcame the drawbacks of short-acting insulin but their longer-acting counterpart did not have 24-hour action; hence, these formulations were not suitable for once-a-day therapy in the majority and were associated with a higher prevalence of hypoglycemia, coformulation of aspart with degludec has very effectively overcome this drawback. Another advantage of this coformulation is that both the components are in solution and retain their individual identity on electrophoresis and also their individual pharmacokinetic properties. Furthermore, there is no need for shaking the formulation before each injection as it is not in suspension form.

Subsequent to the availability of long-acting and ultra-long-acting insulin analogs, ultrarapid-acting versions of aspart (Fiasp) (2018) and lispro (ultrarapid lispro) (2020) were introduced. These analogs get absorbed even quicker as compared to rapid-acting insulin analogs and offer better control of 1-hour postprandial blood glucose levels. In Fiasp niacinamide is added to aspart for further increase in speed of absorption, while in ultrarapid-acting lispro, treprostinil and citrate are added as expedients to facilitate faster absorption. Ultrarapid-acting insulin analog is a small step forward over rapid-acting insulin analogs in the ever-evolving insulin therapy scenario. All the aforementioned insulin analogs except ultrarapid-acting lispro are easily available in India.

■ CONCENTRATED INSULIN

Another direction in which insulin has evolved over the years is the development of concentrated insulin. In patients with severe insulin resistance, injection of large doses of insulin is associated with some disadvantages, such as large volume of injections, which can cause pain or discomfort, and the need for frequent refill prescriptions for insulin vials or pens, which can cause logistic problems. Following insulin products were developed to take care of these problems: (1) U-500 and U-200 short-acting insulin, (2) U-200 degludec, and (3) U-200 lispro. Out of these, U-200 short-acting insulin and U-200 lispro insulin are available in India. All the aforementioned variants have the same pharmacokinetics as those of corresponding U-100 insulin. Formulations with higher concentrations with special manufacturing technology to alter the pharmacokinetics are also available **(Fig. 1)** (glargine 300). In this example, the main purpose of development was to prolong the duration of action.

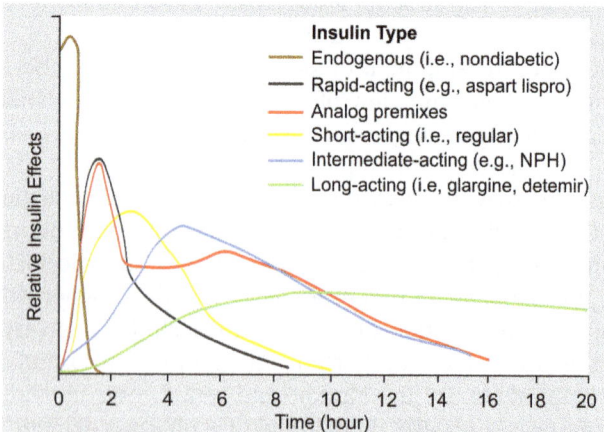

FIG. 1: Pharmacokinetic profiles of human insulin and insulin analogs.

Source: Freeman JS. Insulin analog therapy: improving the match with physiologic insulin secretion. J Am Osteopath Assoc. 2009;109(1):26-36. Quoted by White JR Insulin analogs: what are the clinical implications of structural differences? US Pharm. 2010;35(5)(Diabetes Suppl):3-7.

BIOSIMILAR INSULIN

The ultimate aim of the medical profession is to achieve optimal glycemic control in as many patients as possible. We now have adequate medicines to do this, provided patients are compliant with our prescription. Alas, in reality, noncompliance with prescriptions is rampant, and one of the main reasons is the cost of therapy, particularly modern insulin analog therapy in a country like India, where the majority of the patients buy medicines out of pocket. Biosimilar insulin is a biological product that is highly similar to a reference biological product of a pioneer company that invented it, notwithstanding minor differences in clinically inactive components. There are no clinically meaningful differences between the biosimilar product and the reference product in terms of the safety, purity, and potency of the product. In short biosimilar insulin is more or less an exact copy of approved and thus commonly prescribed insulin from an inventor company, manufactured by a competitor company using its own technology and marketed at a considerably lower cost to the user. Thus, availability of high-quality insulin products at lower cost leads to more compliance with the prescription and thus, better glycemic control. In short biosimilar insulin is similar to a generic drug. Why it is called *biosimilar* and not generic and several other questions are answered in a chapter on biosimilar insulin. Thus, the manufacturing of several biosimilar insulin products, their acceptance by the licensing authorities, and their availability at lower and affordable costs was a major step forward in the evolution of insulin therapy. We should be proud to know that Biocon, a Bengaluru-based biotechnology company has developed biosimilar glargine that is not only available in India but also available in countries including Japan and USA; where it is licensed as interchangeable biosimilar insulin meaning thereby that even if a patient carries prescription for the branded innovator glargine to the chemist's shop, the later has legal rights to replace it with Biocon's glargine without consulting the prescribing doctor. This is a classic example of the success of the *"Atmanirbhar Bharat"* (self-reliance) and "Made in India for the world" policies of the Government of India.

Flowchart 1 gives the timeline for the insulin development.

FUTURE OF INSULIN

Revolution comes in one stroke, introduction of insulin in clinical practice in 1922, revolutionized treatment of diabetes, subsequent continuous and ongoing improvements, in big and or small steps at a time is an ongoing evolution which will ever continue. Now let us take a view of some future insulin products in the pipeline.

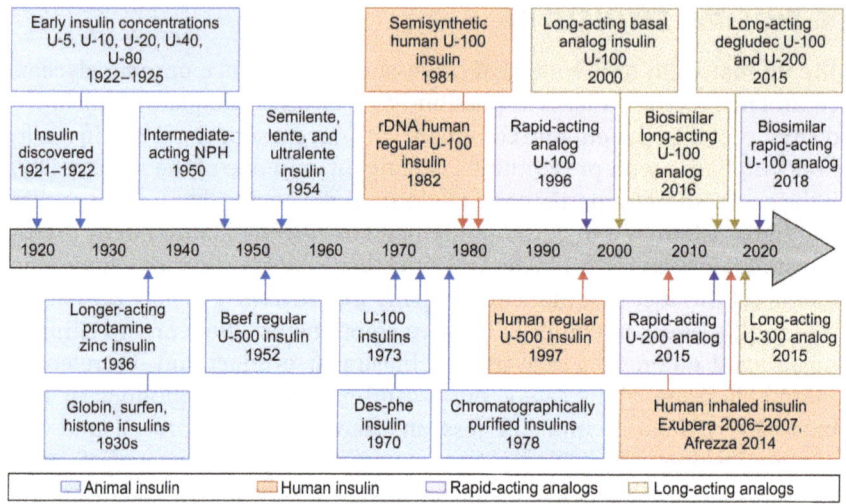

FLOWCHART 1: Timeline of insulin development with approximate historical dates.
(NPH: neutral protamine Hagedorn; rDNA: recombinant deoxyribonucleic acid; U: units)
Source: Hirsch IB, Juneja R, Beals JM, Antalis CJ, Wright EE. The Evolution of Insulin and How it Informs Therapy and Treatment Choices. Endocr Rev. 2020;41(5):733-55.

■ NOVEL INSULIN MOLECULES IN THE PIPELINE

Once Weekly Long-acting Insulin (Icodec)

Icodec is a long-acting insulin for once-a-week administration. It is in an advanced stage of development and has already completed phase 3 studies. In 26 week comparative study of 526 T2DM patients, the glycemic efficacy as judged by reduction in glycated hemoglobin (HbA1c) and time spent in range during continuous glucose monitoring (CGM) was equal to the patients in the comparative group on once or twice a day long-acting insulin analogs (glargine and glargine 300; degludec). The incidence of hypoglycemia was negligible and equal in both groups.

In a similar comparative study done on T1DM patients, glycemic efficacy was similar but the incidence of hypoglycemia was higher in icodec group, probably because of greater day-to-day variability of insulin requirement in T1DM patients.

Availability of once-a-week long-acting insulin is expected to significantly improve acceptance and ease of insulin initiation and long-term compliance.

Glucose-responsive Insulin

This novel concept is in the early stage of development. Glucose-responsive insulin has two separate sites for host receptors, one each for insulin and mannose, Depending upon prevailing blood glucose concentration, insulin is shunted from one to another receptor site for attachment. When blood glucose falls beyond a threshold, more insulin gets attached to mannose receptors, thus less is available for insulin receptors. In this way, hypoglycemia is avoided.

Insulin Analog 327—Liver Specific Insulin

This insulin analog is also in an early developmental stage. It has an albumin-binding side chain, which considerably reduces its binding to insulin receptors while passing through systemic circulation and helps it selectively concentrate in the liver. Thus, it restores the hepatosystemic insulin gradient and reduces episodes of hypoglycemia.

ORAL INSULIN

Insulin molecule being a protein is split up into its constituent amino acids by the enzymes in the upper gastrointestinal (GI) tract before its absorption in the circulation, thus it is totally ineffective when administered by oral route. However, considering the patient's resistance to accepting injectable insulin, several groups are attempting to develop a system of an envelope or a coating that would prevent the digestion of insulin in the upper GI tract and facilitate its absorption in an intact form. An Indian group working for Biocon, a biotechnology and pharmaceutical concern based in Bengaluru, is at the forefront of the development of oral insulin. They have used polymer technology and their oral insulin (IN 105) is in a phase 3 clinical trial. Some groups are working on nanoparticle technology. Both rapid and long-acting oral insulin preparations are being developed. Research has been ongoing for years, but it still has a long way to come to the market.

MISCELLANEOUS NONINJECTABLE INSULIN PREPARATIONS

Looking at the large potential for insulin administration through the noninjecting route due to severe aversion to lifelong injection of insulin, several groups are working to find out the solution. Subcutaneous patches, orally ingested unfolding microneedle devices, and indigestible micro-applicator devices that adhere to the GI wall and deliver the calibrated dose of insulin, are some of the ongoing projects.

SUMMARY

Since its introduction in clinical practice exactly a century ago, there has been continuous ongoing improvement in insulin molecule. In the initial decades, purity of insulin was the focus of attention. This was followed by the introduction of longer-acting insulin. In the eighties, genetically engineered human insulin was introduced into clinical practice, while around the turn of the century, introduction of rapid-acting analogs followed by long-acting analogs was a major milestone in the ever evolving history of the insulin molecule. Simultaneously, there has been continuous and ongoing development as regards insulin delivery devices. Once a week insulin is expected to enter the therapeutic armamentarium in second half of this year. The availability of biosimilar versions of different insulin formulations is also a very encouraging development as more patients will be able to afford it and diabetes therapy will become more inclusive. While transferring the patent for large scale insulin manufacture almost free of cost to Toronto University, Dr Banting made a statement, *"Insulin does not belong to me, it belongs to everybody".* He would have been extremely pleased to know the progress on biosimilar insulin.

CHAPTER 4

Insulin Physiology and Pathophysiology in Diabetes Mellitus

▰ INTRODUCTION

Diabetes mellitus is a disease resulting from insulin deficiency, either actual or relative; and total or partial. Thus, let us briefly review the normal structure and function of insulin; and its physiological role; and pathophysiological defects which lead to insulin deficiency, ultimately leading to the development of diabetes.

▰ INSULIN PHYSIOLOGY

Insulin is secreted and released by β-cells of the islets of Langerhans in pancreas. Islets are scattered throughout the pancreas. Typically, each islet contains about 1,000 cells, 80% of which are β-cells. About 1–2% of pancreatic mass is formed by the β-cells. Islets are surrounded by dense capillary network and receive around 10 times higher capillary blood supply as compared to exocrine pancreatic tissue. This helps toward free exchange of nutrients between β-cells and capillaries, which is vital for swift nutrient-stimulated β-cell signaling for insulin release. Glucose is the principal nutrient involved in signaling insulin release, but other nutrients, such as certain amino acids, fatty acids, and hormones also play a minor role. Insulin is a small protein containing 51 amino acids arranged in two chains which are interlinked with each other by two disulfide bonds. A chain has 21 amino acids while B chain has 30 amino acids **(Fig. 1)**.

Insulin is synthesized in β-cells as preproinsulin which is then internalized into endoplasmic reticulum, from where it travels to Golgi apparatus. In the vesicles of Golgi apparatus, proinsulin is cleaved and insulin and C-peptide are separately released into circulation in 1:1 proportion in response to rising blood glucose. Thus, estimation of plasma C-peptide is a reliable investigation to study β-cell function. Since C-peptide is not present in externally administered insulin, it can estimate β-cell function and the body's natural ability to form and release its own insulin from β-cells in

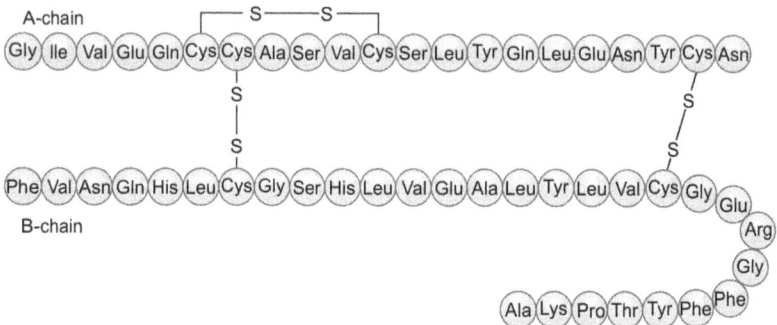

FIG. 1: Structure of human insulin.
Courtesy: (A) OpenStax CNX, under CC by Attribution license; (B) Protein Data Bank (2022).
Source: Morris D. Biosimilar insulins: an in-depth guide. J Diabetes Nurse. 2022;26(1):228.

the pancreas. Insulin is secreted by the β-cells in response to changes in glucose concentrations in a pulsating manner. Rise in plasma glucose, as in postprandial state leads to rise in glucose in β-cells, which is immediately sensed by intracellular glucose transporter 2 (GLUT2) enzyme in β-cells, the process in turns leads to activation of glucokinase, which converts glucose to glucose 6 phosphate, which leads to increase in generation of adenosine triphosphate (ATP), through the intermediary stage of pyruvate formation from glucose 6 phosphate. ATP gets linked to ATP-sensitive potassium channels, which in turn leads to cell membrane depolarization of β-cells and, in turn, opening of calcium channels and entry of extracellular calcium in β-cells. This is the final signal for release of insulin in the circulation **(Fig. 2)**. In the fasting state, which coincides with the basal stage of insulin formation and release, low amplitude insulin pulses are released every 5–6 minutes as per prevailing blood and tissue glucose levels. On an average, 1 unit of insulin is released per hour in portal circulation during the fasting stage. In this stage, insulin levels in portal circulation are 2–5 ng/mL whereas its level in systemic circulation is 0.5 ng/mL. Plasma glucose concentration is maintained by establishing a balance between tissue consumption of glucose and hepatic glucose production. If blood glucose rises, extra insulin is released to suppress hepatic glucose production and if it tends to fall, insulin production is suppressed and glucagon production and release is stimulated, thus hypoglycemia is avoided. In postprandial state, as glucose from digested carbohydrates is absorbed into the circulation, inappropriate rise of blood glucose is prevented by releasing appropriate amount of insulin. Both the frequency and amplitude of insulin pulses are increased **(Fig. 3)**. Postprandially, extra insulin is released in circulation in two phases, a short first phase, which starts in 1–3 minutes and lasts for 10 minutes, and a longer second phase, which starts after about 15 minutes and lasts as long as required to suppress postprandial rise of blood glucose.

CHAPTER 4: Insulin Physiology and Pathophysiology in Diabetes Mellitus

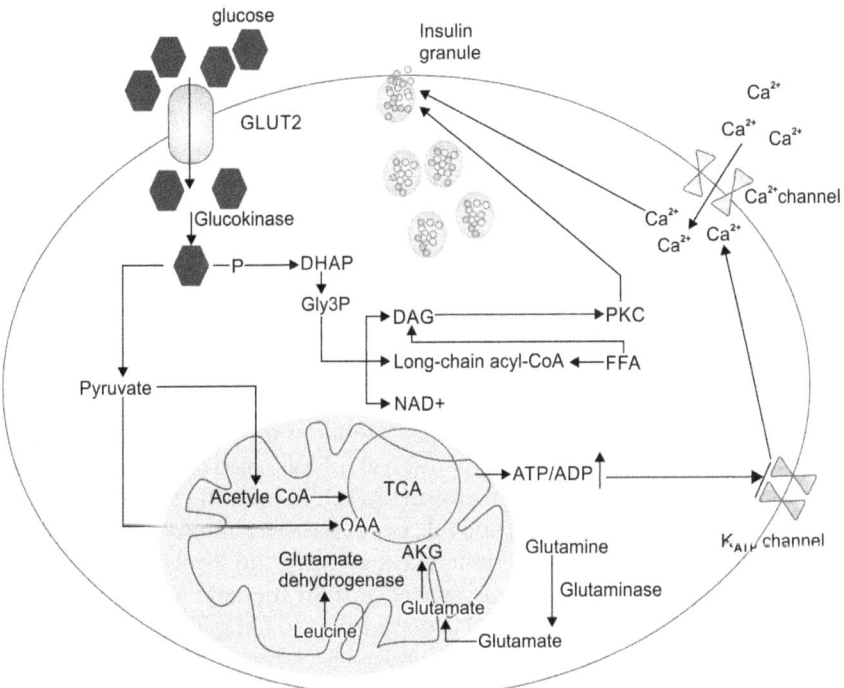

FIG. 2: Schematic representation of nutrient-related insulin release.
(ADP: adenosine diphosphate; AKG: alpha-ketoglutarate; ATP: adenosine triphosphate; CoA: coenzyme A; DAG: diacylglycerol; DHAP: dihydroxyacetone phosphate; FFA: free fatty acids; GLUT2: glucose transporter 2; OAA: oxaloacetate; PKC: protein kinase C; TCA: tricarboxylic acid)
Source: Fu Z, Gilbert ER, Liu D. Regulation of insulin synthesis and secretion and pancreatic Beta-cell dysfunction in diabetes. Curr Diabetes Rev. 2013;9(1):25-53.

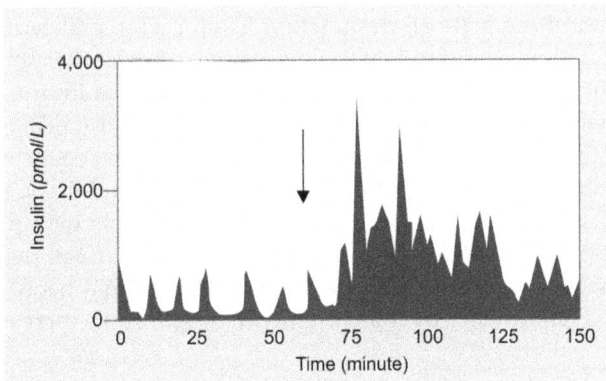

FIG. 3: Pulsatile insulin secretion. Time in minutes on the X-axis and plasma insulin levels on the Y-axis. Downward pointing arrow in the center indicates time of food intake.
Note: Low amplitude relatively infrequent insulin pulses in fasting state in left half of the cartoon and high amplitude frequent pulses in right half during postprandial period.

Insulin is released directly into the portal vein from where 50% of it is extracted for local action during the first pass through the liver. Insulin is an important anabolic hormone with profound action over carbohydrate, protein as well as fat metabolism, and growth promotion. Insulin carries out its activities by combining with insulin receptors situated on cell membranes. Combination of insulin with the extracellular part of insulin receptor leads to generation of downstream signals for its metabolic and growth promotional activities in cytoplasm.

■ PATHOPHYSIOLOGY OF INSULIN SECRETION

In type 1 diabetes mellitus (T1DM), β-cells are completely destroyed by autoimmune process, usually in rapid manner in children, adolescents, and young adults, or in a gradual manner extending over several months, in a subtype of T1DM which is more common in middle-aged people and is called latent autoimmune diabetes in adults (LADA). In both the subgroups, there is hardly any insulin synthesis and release, and these patients require lifelong insulin therapy for survival. Their plasma C-peptide levels are negligible, even in those who have already started insulin therapy. In many cases of LADA, there could be low normal C-peptide levels at the diagnosis and these patients are very likely to be miss diagnosed as patients with type 2 diabetes mellitus (T2DM). Relatively poor response to oral antidiabetic drugs (OADs) from the beginning, which further deteriorates rapidly, and is associated with rapidly reducing C-peptide levels in these patients. The diagnosis is established retrospectively in many of them after months of failed treatment. Established T1DM patients are dependent on externally administered insulin for their survival. In such patients, the discontinuation of insulin will lead to severe metabolic disturbances, terminating into diabetic ketoacidosis and coma, and ultimately death.

In T2DM, there is β-cell dysfunction leading to insufficient first phase insulin secretion and gradually diminishing overall insulin secretion. In addition to the insulin secretory β-cell defects, significant majority of T2DM patients also have varying degrees of insulin resistance, mainly from adoption of faulty lifestyle sometimes superadded with genetic component, which is usually polygenic. In these patients, peripheral tissue response to available insulin is less than normal. These patients also have postprandial incretin hormone deficiency. In addition, there is an α-cell defect leading to inappropriate high secretion of glucagon (in normal people, glucagon secretion is controlled by blood glucose level. It is increased during

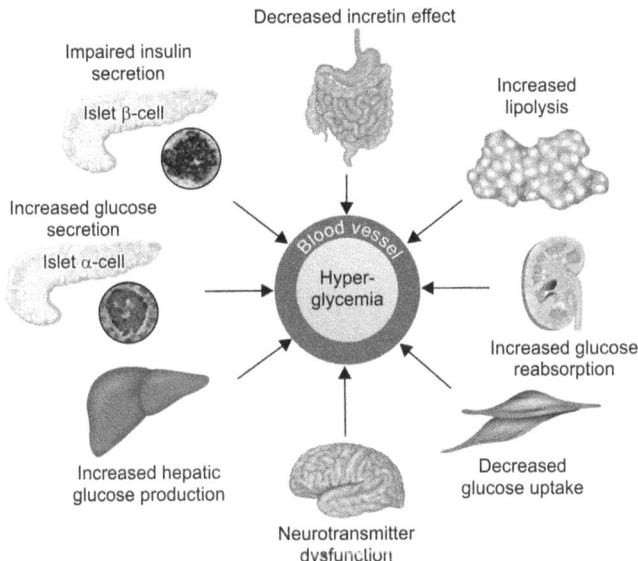

FIG. 4: Sites of pathophysiological defects contributing to hyperglycemia in type 2 diabetes mellitus.
Source: Defronzo RA. Banting Lecture. From the triumvirate to the ominous octet: a new paradigm for the treatment of type 2 diabetes mellitus. Diabetes. 2009;58(4):773-95.

hypoglycemia and suppressed during hyperglycemia) **(Fig. 4)**. These additional defects put ever increasing load on β-cells to produce extra insulin to overdrive them and maintain glycemic balance. Those with limited β-cell capacity due to genetic and/or acquired β-cell insufficiency, fail to fulfill ever increasing demand at some point, leading to the onset of diabetes mellitus which progresses further. Most of the T2DM patients have varying degrees of these defects; however, till they reach "end stage β-cell failure", they retain the capacity to produce varying amounts of endogenous insulin which, even though not sufficient to control blood glucose, is sufficient to prevent diabetic ketoacidosis. T2DM patients are not dependent on insulin for survival; thus, they were classified as noninsulin-dependent diabetics in the past. However, over the years, the capacity of their β-cells gradually diminishes and a time will come when they cannot be controlled by oral pills and/or glucagon-like peptide-1 receptor agonists (GLP-1 RAs) any longer, even if all the major classes are combined together. At this stage, they require insulin to achieve blood glucose control **(Fig. 5)**.

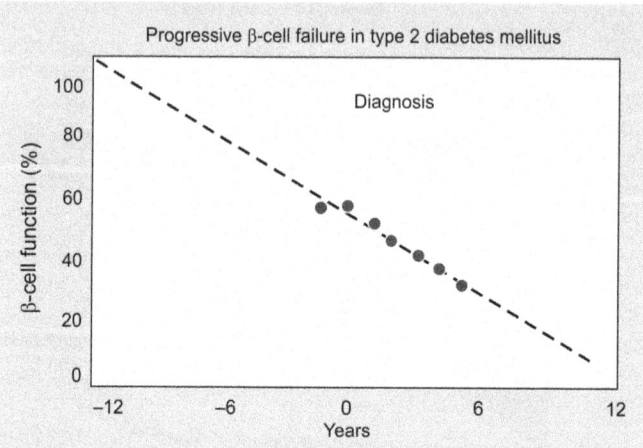

FIG. 5: Duration of diabetes in years on the X-axis (time of diagnosis of diabetes is zero years); and the functional capacity of β-cells for insulin secretion and release on Y-axis.

Source: Adapted from U.K. prospective diabetes study 16. Overview of 6 years' therapy of type 2 diabetes: a progressive disease. U.K. Prospective Diabetes Study Group. Diabetes. 1995;44(11):1249-58. Erratum in: Diabetes. 1996;45(11):1655.

Note following points:
- Functional capacity of β-cells starts to gradually reduce several years before the onset of and obviously before the diagnosis of type 2 diabetes mellitus.
- At the time of diagnosis, which could be delayed for up to 5 years after the onset, the functional capacity of β-cells is around 50% and is on continuous ongoing decline.
- Several years after the diagnosis, the functional capacity of β-cells could be negligible.

SUMMARY

Insulin is a vital hormone secreted by β cells situated in islets of Langerhans in the pancreas. It has profound effects on metabolism of carbohydrates, proteins; and fats and in addition, it has anabolic properties. Insulin deficiency, eighter complete, or partial and relative, is essential for the development of diabetes. Besides pancreas, several pathophysiological defects in different organs are responsible for metabolic derangement which leads to relative insulin deficiency in T2DM. In the management of hyperglycemia, externally administered insulin has the highest therapeutic value and, unlike all other antidiabetic agents, it has no contraindications. It works in all types of diabetes and in all the stages of diabetes. Like any other therapeutic agent, it has some limitations and side effects, which are principally due to the unphysiological route of administration of insulin in the subcutaneous tissue, which one has to resort to.

CHAPTER 5

Biosimilar Insulin

INTRODUCTION

It is expected that like other biosimilar drugs such as sera, vaccines, hormones, etc., affordably priced biosimilar insulin will play more active role in the management of diabetes. Thus, the subject of biosimilar insulin attains significance. Let us understand basics of biosimilar drugs.

BIOLOGICAL DRUGS OR BIOLOGICALS

Drugs or therapeutic agents which we use in our clinical practice are basically divided into two different classes. (1) Drugs with a simple chemical structure having a low molecular weight, e.g., metformin; and (2) High molecular weight complex protein-based drugs which are usually manufactured by using live microorganisms and employing biotechnology, e.g., vaccines, immunoglobulins, immunomodulators, immunosuppressants, insulin, including insulin analogs, etc. Healthcare-related sciences such as microbiology, virology, immunology, clinical and paraclinical sciences, pharmaceutical sciences are all progressing at rapid rate and as a result more and more previously untreatable or inadequately treatable disorders are now having therapeutic solutions, often in the form of complex biological medicines. The research and development and manufacturing of biological drugs involve complex, high technology, cost-intensive and time-consuming processes. Thus, biological medicines are usually very expensive, particularly during initial exclusivity period during which, to enable the innovator to recover the cost of research and development and to encourage future development of new innovative drug entities, a competitor is not allowed to introduce a copy of same drug in the market. Unlike a simple chemical drug, a copy of innovator drug introduced in the market by a competitor is not called a generic drug, but is called a biosimilar drug. So, let us find out exact meaning of a biosimilar drug and how does it differ from generic drug.

BIOSIMILAR MEDICINE

A biosimilar medicine is a copy version of an existing approved biological medicine. It is defined as a biological medicine that has no clinically meaningful difference with the originator molecule in terms of quality, safety, efficacy, or immunogenicity [European Medicines Agency (EMA), 2014a; NHS England, 2019]. Implicit in the definition of biosimilar medicine is that its structure need not exactly match the original product, but clinical efficacy and safety profile should exactly match the original product of innovator company. The generic drug is defined as chemically synthesized small molecule drug using the same active ingredient, dosage form, route of administration, conditions of use as the reference product. For example, Diamicron is innovator's brand of gliclazide, while Cyblex, Glizid, etc., are generic versions of gliclazide in India. Since they are also branded, they are called branded generics. When generics are sold under chemical name, they are called generics. In advanced countries, generics are usually marketed under chemical names and are called (just plain) generics; however, biosimilars usually carry trade names. Lantus is branded glargine of an innovator company and Basalog is branded biosimilar drug made available by Biocon of India in several international markets as well as in India. So, Basalog is branded biosimilar insulin. The intention of encouraging introduction of biosimilar medicines in the market is to reduce the cost of medicine so that more patients can be treated with them.

Why Biosimilar Insulins may not be and Need not be Exact Copies of Innovator Insulin?

The intricate manufacturing process adapted by the manufacturer of biosimilar medicines including insulin is different as compared to the innovator. In case of insulin, a different microorganism (e.g., *Escherichia coli* in place of *Saccharomyces*), or different strain of same organism can be used. Sometimes a strain of same microorganism can show some minor variation from batch to batch, thus, even an innovator brand can have minor changes from batch to batch. These factors are likely to lead to small differences between the biosimilar and its originator. However, safety and efficacy of biosimilar have to be identical with that of innovator brand.

What is Interchangeable Insulin?

Recently, Food and Drug Administration (FDA), the drug regulatory authority of USA introduced rules regarding interchangeability of biosimilar insulin. Basaglar, the biosimilar brand of glargine, manufactured by Bengaluru-based Biocon Biologics Ltd., which was already approved by FDA in 2020 for its biosimilarity to glargine, was the first biosimilar insulin to receive interchangeability status in USA in 2021.

It is to be noted that all biosimilar insulins are not automatically interchangeable. If a prescribing doctor wants to start glargine in a particular patient, he can prescribe innovator's glargine or biosimilar glargine and a chemist has to dispense whatever glargine the doctor has prescribed, he cannot replace the insulin at his level. But, if the biosimilar insulin has received certificate of interchangeability from the regulatory authority, chemist has the choice of dispensing either innovator's brand or interchangeable insulin, without consulting the prescribing doctor. Obviously for biosimilar insulin to become interchangeable insulin, additional analytical and clinical trial data have to be submitted for thorough scrutiny.

Availability of More Biosimilar Brands of Insulin is the Need of the Day

Diabetes is the disease resulting from insulin deficiency. In type 1 diabetes mellitus (T1DM), life is not possible without insulin. In type 2 diabetes mellitus (T2DM), progressive insulin deficiency often drives metabolic derangements and thus, in spite of availability of new groups of medications such as dipeptidyl peptidase-4 (DPP-4) inhibitors, glucagon-like peptide-1 receptor agonists (GLP-1 RAs), and sodium-glucose cotransporter-2 (SGLT-2) inhibitors, majority of patients require insulin for glycemic control some years after the onset of diabetes. Though, introduction of insulin can be postponed, it cannot be avoided. Tight metabolic control is essential to prevent complications of diabetes and to improve quality of life and longevity. The availability, accessibility, and affordability of insulin are vitally important. Like most other biological drugs, insulin is expensive, and the high cost of insulin is one of the main reasons responsible for patient's noncomplaince with insulin thus, availability of biosimilar insulin at affordable cost is vitally important. Biosimilar insulins are about 35% less expensive than innovator brands. However, since manufacturing of biological drugs like insulin involves high technology, infrastructure, expertise, knowledge, and large-scale investment and long incubation period. Furthermore, as compared to getting licenses to manufacture and subsequently market chemical drugs, insulin requires a lot of mandatory analytical, phase 1 and phase III testing which again is time-consuming and expensive. Thus, manufacture of products like insulin can only be undertaken by large biological companies and not by micro- or small-scale chemical companies operating from small units in industrial estates. A quick google search identified >600 and 300 generic metformin and glimepiride brands in India respectively, but biosimilar brands of insulin can be counted on fingers of one hand. The situation is similar even in advanced countries such as USA and European Union, particularly for biosimilar insulin, though it is somewhat better for other biosimilar products, as regards number of biosimilar drugs but not regards number of biosimilar copies of the same drug. Thus, the difference between the cost of innovator drug and biosimilar copies is not as big as that between the cost of innovator brand of a small molecular weight chemical drug and its generic copies. If availability of insulin needs to be drastically improved, then regulatory government authorities, drug industry, medical profession, and nongovernmental organization (NGO) groups looking after patients' interest, all should come together to find out ways and means of reducing cost of insulin. Encouraging more companies to manufacture biosimilar insulin, so that 5-6 brands of each insulin are available in market to start with is one of the ways to achieve the goal of drastically increasing affordability, availability, and accessibility of insulin. Of course, ensuring high quality of all the biosimilar brands will be equally important. The author foresees a very small number of high technology companies having the expertise to manufacture insulin will supply biosimilar insulin to a large number of marketing companies which would brand the biosimilar insulin and market it. Even such activity will introduce healthy competition which will definitely lead to reduction of the cost of insulin. Looking at the number of companies with major and successful presence in oral antidiabetic medications market, who have recently introduced biosimilar glargine as well as biosimilar human insulin in recent past, the trend has definitely gathered speed in last 12 months. The success of these biosimilar insulins will lead to more high technology biological companies entering the market.

SUMMARY

Insulin is a complex high molecular weight protein and, like other biological products such as sera and vaccines, is manufactured by a biological process involving genetic engineering technology. Thus, inventing alternative process for mass manufacturing is time consuming and involves high technology and cost. This is the main reason for the paucity of bio similar drugs, which are biological equivalents of generic chemical drugs, in our armamentarium. However, for any new therapeutic intervention to be really effective at a level of larger society, should be affordable to the people in lower economical strata of the society. Thus, availability of biosimilar alternatives to as many biological drugs as possible and more than one alternative for each biological drug, including insulin, is the need of the day. Recent developments in the field of biosimilar insulin is a step in the right direction.

CHAPTER 6

Insulin Resistance

■ INTRODUCTION

Insulin resistance (IR) has many definitions. The most commonly accepted and clinically oriented definition is as follows: IR is a pathophysiological state in which there is a resistance from the tissues, such as muscles, fat, and liver to the physiological actions of insulin, resulting in to reduced effect of insulin. Insulin carries out two different physiological functions, namely, (1) acute metabolic functions such as glucose regulation and (2) long-term functions on tissue growth and proliferation. These two sets of actions are carried out through activating two different sets of insulin receptors. Conventionally, the term IR includes resistance to acute effects of insulin resulting in deranged carbohydrate metabolism. Diabetic patients requiring >1 unit of insulin/kg of their body weight per day are called insulin resistant and those requiring >200 U/day are considered as having severe IR. However, this definition has obvious limitations as it excludes nondiabetic insulin resistant people and also those diabetics who are not taking insulin.

■ ETIOLOGY OF INSULIN RESISTANCE

Several genetic and acquired causes lead to IR. While specific monogenic defects leading to IR are associated with rare syndromes such as Leprechaunism and Rabson–Mendenhall syndrome, the common type of IR which one comes across in a day-to-day practice is one that results from interplay between acquired causes with some contribution from underlying genetic defects which are usually polygenic. In this concise practical handbook, which is specifically written for primary and secondary care physicians and resident doctors to help them to make bedside decisions related to insulin therapy in their day-to-day practice, we will be mainly covering the clinical and therapeutic aspects of common type of IR which a clinician comes across routinely in a day-to-day practice and thus will use the clinical definition of IR. *Thus, IR is a state in which a given increase in plasma insulin level in the affected individual causes less of an effect on lowering the glucose level than it does in a normal individual*

Insulin resistance and diabetes, particularly type 2 diabetes mellitus (T2DM), are not synonymous, but they almost always overlap in a given individual and contribute together toward glycemic derangement and resultant cascading metabolic and vascular derangement. Though, it is difficult to identify which developed first in a given individual, more often IR precedes T2DM. Every individual having IR does not develop T2DM, similarly every patient having T2DM does not have significant IR, though most have some degree of contribution from IR toward hyperglycemia, varying from minimum to dominant contribution.

The principle physiological actions of insulin include control of plasma glucose level by preventing excessive formation of glucose in the liver by controlling the breakdown of stored glycogen into glucose (glycogenolysis) and also by preventing conversion of amino acids in to glucose (neoglucogenesis); and by facilitating entry of glucose into tissues such as muscles from plasma. In a patient with IR, reduced efficiency of both the aforementioned processes tends to increase in plasma glucose level, which is immediately sensed by glucokinase sensors and the signal is transmitted to the β-cells in islets of Langerhans in pancreas to synthesize and release more insulin to counteract its reduced efficiency due to IR. Thus, as long as the β-cells have the capacity to respond to increased demand to synthesize and release more insulin, plasma glucose level is maintained in normal range but at the cost of extra workload on the β-cells and resultant hyperinsulinemia Thus, in those with healthy β-cells, IR does not automatically and immediately lead to T2DM as long as the β-cells have the capacity to respond to extra demand on insulin. This explains why all people with IR are not necessarily diabetic. In those who have genetic defects leading to limited β-cell capacity, usually due to multiple gene involvement, with or without additional acquired causes such as faulty lifestyle leading to obesity, the capacity to respond to extra demand on insulin is limited. In such a situation, if IR persists or increases in severity (though IR can be partly reduced by appropriately tackling acquired causes), a time comes when chronic extra work load gradually leads to exhaustion of β-cells, leading to inability to meet the ever-increasing demand for more insulin. At this stage, prediabetes develops and the persistence of IR subsequently leads to development of T2DM **(Fig. 1)**.

PREVALENCE OF INSULIN RESISTANCE

It is estimated that about 25% of the population is insulin resistant, thus the prevalence of IR is roughly twice as compared to that of T2DM. IR is present in 65–75% of those with impaired glucose tolerance and in about 85% of T2DM patients.

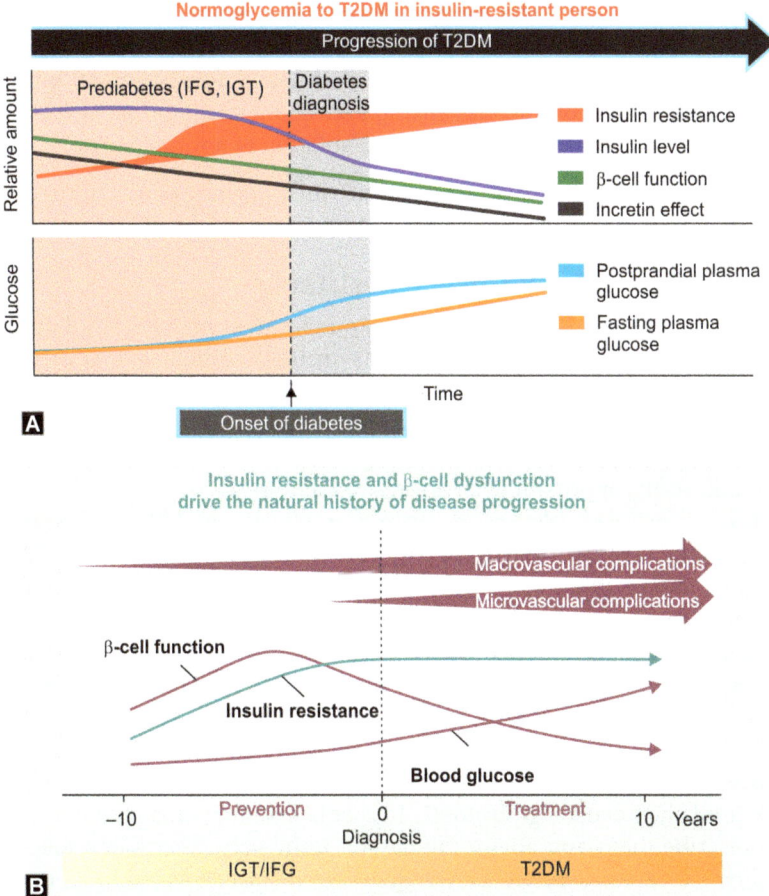

FIGS. 1A AND B: Natural history of progression of normoglycemia to T2DM with insulin resistance.
(IGF: impaired fasting glucose; IGT: impaired glucose tolerance; T2DM: type 2 diabetes mellitus)
Sources: (A) Kendall DM, Cuddihy RM, Bergenstal RM. Clinical application of incretin-based therapy: therapeutic potential, patient selection and clinical use. Am J Med. 2009;122(6 Suppl):S37-50. (B) DeFronzo RA. Pathogenesis of type 2 diabetes mellitus. Med Clin North Am. 2004;88(4):787-835, ix.

Methods of Estimation of Insulin Resistance

There are several methods to assess IR. All the methods assess the relationship between plasma glucose and plasma insulin. While the gold standard is euglycemic-hyperinsulinemic clamp study, this method is time-consuming and difficult to perform in a day-to-day clinical setting. The most commonly performed method in clinical practice is homeostatic model assessment (HOMA). This method is simple and only requires measurement of fasting plasma glucose and insulin levels. HOMA is based on a computer program derived assessment of the relationship between fasting plasma glucose and fasting plasma insulin levels in a large population of normal persons.

$$\text{HOMA IR} = \text{fasting plasma insulin } (\mu U/mL) \times \text{fasting plasma glucose (mmol/L)}/22.5$$

Bedside Tips to Tackle Insulin Resistance

- Lifestyle management is the cornerstone for treatment of IR. All diabetic patients need a thorough education on lifestyle management through diet and exercise. Emphasis should be placed on implementation and reaching the waist circumference and weight goals. Also look for drug-induced obesity (e.g., antidepressants) and look for alternative medications or possibility of dosage reduction.
- Take a detailed history of current medications. Many patients are simultaneously treated by more than one doctor. It is possible that your patient is under a dermatologist for allergic skin conditions or under another doctor who is treating his "asthma". Under both the aforementioned circumstances, he is likely to be taking corticosteroids without your knowledge. Thiazide diuretics such as hydrochlorothiazide, statins, and β-blockers are some of the common drugs which can increase IR. Whenever an alternative drug is available, prefer it. If it is not available, use it in minimum effective dose, e.g., up to 12.5 mg of hydrochlorothiazide is unlikely to cause significant IR. In case of essential drugs such as statins, prescribe them and advise the patient to be very strict about following diet and exercise and reach weight goals. In case of steroids, do not use them in indications where their role is empirical and when they are essential, adjust the dose of antidiabetics to maintain glycemic control. Most diabetic patients on moderate-to-high doses of steroids will need insulin for good glycemic control, even if they were at their glycemic goals before starting steroids.
- Carefully search for occult infections such as urinary tract infections and tuberculosis by taking detailed history and ordering appropriate investigations. Many infections cause IR and control of infection leads to reversal of IR to preinfection level.
- Choose the right antidiabetic medicines. Sodium-glucose cotransporter-2 (SGLT-2) inhibitors and glucagon-like peptide-1 receptor agonists (GLP-1 RAs) are associated with significant weight loss and both the groups offer cardio and renal protection. These agents should be judiciously used in day-to-day practice. Suitable grossly overweight patients should be offered metabolic surgery.
- Insulin-induced hypoglycemia and fear of insulin-induced hypoglycemia are important weight gain inducing factors. Thus, judiciously select

insulin preparation to minimize hypoglycemic episodes (e.g., long-acting insulin analogs and rapid-acting insulin analogs in place of intermediate-acting and short-acting insulin) in appropriate patients. Judiciously uptitrate insulin when required, avoid sliding scale method. This will help to minimize iatrogenic therapeutic hyperinsulinemia and reduce weight gain.

SUMMARY

Insulin resistance is a common condition and is commonly associated with T2DM, in whom it worsens glycemic control, leads to increased requirement for antidiabetic medications and is a driving pathophysiological factor responsible for increased prevalence of diseases such as atherosclerotic cardiovascular disorders (ASCVDs), hypertension, obesity, nonalcoholic fatty liver disease, etc. Thus, during every consultation with the patients, efforts should be made towards assessment and management of IR. Remember, ASCVD is responsible for two-thirds of deaths as well as reduced longevity in patients with T2DM and the driving factor for acceleration of ASCVD in diabetes is associated IR. So strike it with full force to improve diabetic patient's longevity and quality of life, do not have glucocentric approach.

PSYCHOLOGICAL INSULIN RESISTANCE

All patients with type 1 diabetes mellitus (T1DM) require insulin for survival and patients or their parents grasp this fact and reluctantly accept insulin. So, let us keep this subtype of diabetes out of discussion as far as psychological insulin resistance (PIR) is concerned and concentrate on type 2 diabetes mellitus (T2DM), which is a progressive disease and thus, at some point of their journey with the disease, majority will require insulin to maintain glycemic control, if not for immediate survival. However, their long-term survival is at stake if they do not accept insulin and thus have poor glycemic control over a long term. This fact is poorly understood and whenever their doctor advises insulin, many reject the advice. *PIR is defined as opposition toward insulin use or rejection of idea of insulin use.* Many studies quoted in the literature estimate the prevalence of PIR to be about 30–33%, though in my personal diabetes practice, I found it much higher. In India, average time taken by the patient to start insulin therapy is about 9 years after it became necessary for glycemic control, and thus, average HbA1c when they finally accept insulin is around 9%. Thus, it is not surprising at all that prevalence of various vascular and infective complications of diabetes is far higher than in patients treated in developed countries and having comparative duration of diabetes. Many psychological factors are responsible for PIR, these include:
- Fear of insulin injections and pain at the time of injection
- Fear of hypoglycemia and/or weight gain

- Lack of confidence for mastering self-injection technique
- Fear of dependence on insulin for a lifetime
- Fear of living a restrictive life
- Doubt about ability of insulin to help achieve glycemic targets
- Guilt that he has failed to manage his diabetes and the misconception that he has come toward the end of his life.
- Perception that insulin is a punishment.
- Many patients with PIR have multiple factors operating together.

PSYCHOLOGICAL INSULIN RESISTANCE IN CLINICIAN'S MIND

The majority of patients with diabetes are treated by primary care physicians, many of them with qualifications from alternative system of medicine. Some doctors have PIR, for reasons such as:
- Patients will not be able to manage insulin.
- Patients will leave him and go to another doctor forever.
- Patients will have a high prevalence of hypoglycemia and blame the prescribing doctor.
- Doctor's work will be overloaded by repeated queries.
- Doctor's lack of in-depth knowledge to prescribe correct insulin in correct dosages and when and how to intensify insulin
- Physicians PIR is often referred to as physicians inertia. Physician inertia is defined as failure of a physician to initiate or intensify insulin therapy when necessary or ability to recognize the problem but failure to act.

MANAGEMENT OF PSYCHOLOGICAL INSULIN RESISTANCE

Psychological insulin resistance is a major obstacle in the path of diabetic patients reaching their glycemic goals. Thus, they are exposed to complications of diabetes which reduce their longevity, hamper their quality of life, and make them dependent on others. Thus, the problem of PIR needs to be tackled on a war footing. The treating physician needs to analyze the patient's perceptions and misconceptions in detail and find out which among the aforementioned objections are the main reasons for PIR. Subsequently, detailed education, curated to his individual requirements, should be given.

During the interactions, doctors should show empathy and as far as possible, use the language preferred by the patient and talk at the level meeting the patient's wavelength. Insulin conversation should be initiated at first consultation itself, even though at that point of time many will not require insulin. Some basic information on Insulin and its normal role in the human body and how it is different from other drugs which are synthetic and manufactured in a chemical factory, should be given to the patient and repeated periodically during the follow-up visits. Information on insulin should be projected in a positive manner and advising it in a threatening manner should be strictly avoided. Some patients prefer one to one talk, while others are more comfortable in an informal group discussion where they can interact with other patients who have similar problems or have gone through them. In some situations, audiovisual media can be used. During the interactions, direct questions should be avoided and maximum information should be sought from the patients by asking indirect questions and making them open up their mind. Live demonstrations should be used to convince the patients about the ease of administration of insulin and the lack of any significant pain. Demonstrating insulin pen and syringe with an attached small and delicate needle itself convinces some patients about the unlikelihood of significant pain. A more convincing way is to take an injection of normal saline from an insulin syringe in front of the patient. PIR in minds of primary care physicians should be tackled by providing periodic educational inputs on practical aspects of use of insulin in the management of diabetes through physical and virtual conference and symposia.

■ SUMMARY

Psychological insulin resistance is very common and is a major stumbling block in the way of patients reaching their glycemic goals. It is an "elephant in the room", everybody is aware of it but still shove it under the carpet for various reasons such as lack of time at the doctor's disposal and PIR in doctor's mind. Unless the patient starts taking insulin and adheres to it as per the doctor's advice, he is not going to reach the glycemic goals and avoid the dreaded complications of diabetes. Mere insulin prescription does not help beyond giving legal protection to the prescribing doctor. Thus, every clinician should develop conversational skills and ability to convince the patients about starting insulin as soon as it is required, and should make provision for time required to remove PIR from patient's mind, to attain glycemic control. It is hoped that the medical profession will be able to gainfully translate the rapid strides made in the fields of science and technology to overcome PIR. With rapid and long-acting analogs, objections regarding hypoglycemia and weight gain can be tackled in a better way and with the user-friendly insulin pens, objections regarding pain at the time of injection and lack of discreteness while injecting can be tackled more effectively. Similarly, one can gainfully utilize massive advances in communication systems to spread knowledge and remove misconceptions and objections about insulin therapy.

CHAPTER 7

Insulin in the Management of Diabetes

INTRODUCTION

Diabetes is a lifelong disease with high mortality and morbidity, mainly through macrovascular and microvascular complications. The only way to prevent, postpone, or slow down the rate of progression of microvascular complications is to achieve persistent tight control of blood glucose levels. The major clinical trials [DCCT (Diabetes Control and Complication Trial) in type 1 diabetes and UKPDS (United Kingdom Prospective Diabetes Study) in type 2 diabetes] have proved the importance of appropriately aggressive treatment. In type 1 diabetes, intensive therapy can reduce the incidence of microvascular complications by up to 60% while the reduction is less impressive in type 2 diabetes only because, in some patients, by the time diagnosis of diabetes is established, complications have already set in. In our pursuit to achieve the glycemic and other targets, we must aggressively manage diabetes by judiciously utilizing all the modalities of management namely diet, exercise, and medications including insulin in a coordinated manner. Insulin is a must in all type 1 diabetics and at any point in a busy diabetic clinic; about 33% of type 2 diabetics would require insulin to achieve the goal of tight blood glucose control. A clinician should be very well versed with knowledge about when to start insulin in type 2 diabetes and an even more vital requirement is to acquire the skill to convince the patient to accept insulin without any delay, once a clinician has made up his mind about the need of insulin in a particular patient. Aggressive management and tight blood glucose control are also associated with a higher prevalence of hypoglycemic episodes. Thus, insulin and other antidiabetic agents should be used judiciously.

GLYCEMIC GOALS

Goals for ambulatory patients are enumerated in **Table 1**.
Goals for hospitalized patients are enumerated in **Table 2**.

CHAPTER 7: Insulin in the Management of Diabetes

TABLE 1: Goals for ambulatory patients.

Parameter	AACE	IDF	ADA
HbA1c (%)	<6.5	<6.5	<7.0
Fasting/premeal glucose (mg%)	<110	<100	80–130
Postmeal glucose (mg%)	<140	<160	<180

(AACE: American Association of Clinical Endocrinologists; ADA: American Diabetes Association; HbA1c: glycated hemoglobin; IDF: International Diabetes Federation)

TABLE 2: Goals for hospitalized patients.

Level of care	Glycemic targets in mg%
ICU	• 140–180 • More stringent goals such as 110–140 may be appropriate for selected patients, e.g., after CABG
Non-ICU	• Fasting 80–120 • Premeal < 140 • Postmeal < 180

(CABG: coronary artery bypass grafting; ICU: intensive care unit)

Note: These are general guidelines. Depending upon ground realities in a given patient, one needs to set individualized goals.

Till the eighties, we had only bovine insulin and practically only one brand of insulin. Moreover, it was available in only one strength, 40 units/mL. New developments have taken place in the field of insulin therapy over the last four decades at a rapid rate. Bovine insulin and subsequently introduced porcine insulin has virtually become extinct and totally replaced by human insulin and analogs of human insulin. Human insulin is manufactured by genetic engineering technology, which has virtually eliminated raw material shortages. We also have ready-made insulin mixtures in different proportions. We have a choice of two different strengths of insulin and also have a choice regarding insulin administration devices due to the availability of patient-friendly insulin pens. We also have several designer insulin analogs such as lispro insulin, insulin aspart, Fiasp (ultrarapid-acting insulin), glargine, detemir, degludec, and glargine 300. Thus, besides deciding when to use insulin and in what dosage schedule, a practitioner now has to make several decisions such as which strength? Which device? When to use rapid-acting and long-acting insulin analogs? How to achieve good metabolic control without significantly increasing hypoglycemic episodes? Thus, he needs to regularly update his knowledge to keep pace with the availability of innovative newer insulin preparations at a rapid rate and also with the availability of scientific information.

■ INSULIN PHARMACOLOGY

On the basis of onset of action and duration of action, the insulin preparations available in the market are divided in the categories enumerated here.

Short-acting Insulin

Short-acting insulin is also called regular, clear, or crystalline insulin and was previously available in bovine, porcine as well as human forms in our country; however, human insulin has virtually replaced both the varieties of animal insulin. It is used for the control of postprandial rise in blood glucose levels. Regular human insulin has an onset of action in 30–60 minutes, peak action between 2 and 3 hours, and duration of effective action for 3–6 hours; however, there are many variations from patient to patient. Short-acting insulin is usually used in combination with intermediate-acting or long-acting insulin. In many type 1 diabetics and type 2 diabetics, after having reached the stage of β-cell failure, short-acting insulin is required before each major meal to control postprandial hyperglycemia. However, short-acting insulin administered before dinner is unlikely to control the next morning's fasting blood glucose (FBG), while the shot administered before lunch is unlikely to be effective till dinner. Intermediate or long-acting insulin administered concurrently along with short-acting insulin takes over at these times by providing basal insulinization. In order to effectively suppress postprandial rise in blood glucose levels, short-acting insulin should be injected 30 minutes before meals. Often, in a day-to-day practice either this instruction is not conveyed to the patient or he does not understand it or ignores it and injects insulin just before meals. Such action can lead to poor postprandial control and in pursuit of improving postprandial glucose; insulin dose is often increased without paying attention to the timing of insulin injection. This can lead to late postprandial hypoglycemia. The short-acting insulin available in the market is genetically engineered human insulin having exactly the same structure as native human insulin secreted by β-cells in the pancreas. It has two amino acid chains, A chain with 21 amino acids and B chain with 30 amino acids, connected to each other with two disulfide bonds.

Short-acting insulin is usually administered along with long-acting insulin or intermediate-acting insulin as a prandial component of basal-bolus insulin therapy. In full-fledged basal bolus therapy, it is given before each meal, thus, usually three times a day. In less intensive basal-bolus therapies, it is given before one to two meals, leaving a meal or two with acceptable postprandial blood glucose rise, uncovered.

Rapid-acting Insulin Analogs

Insulin analogs are especially designed insulin in which the amino acid sequence of native human insulin is altered to get a favorable pharmacokinetic profile, without altering the biological activity of insulin. The rapid-acting insulin analogs available in India are lispro insulin,

insulin aspart, and glulisine. Lispro insulin happens to be the first marketed insulin analog. In lispro insulin, amino acids at positions B28 and B29 are interchanged. It has an onset of action in 15–30 minutes, peak action between 30 and 90 minutes after administration, and an effective duration of action of 3–4 hours. In insulin aspart, proline at B28 is replaced by aspartic acid. This alters the pharmacokinetic profile which is similar to that of lispro. Glulisine is manufactured by replacing asparagine with lysine at the B3 position and lysine with glutamic acid at the B26 position. Refer to **Figures 1A to C** for structure of rapid acting insulin. Its pharmacokinetic profile is similar to that of lispro and aspart insulin. Lispro, aspart, or glulisine insulin should be used in place of short-acting insulin in those patients in whom short-acting insulin is unable to control postprandial blood glucose peaks or its use leads to late postprandial hypoglycemia. Another advantage of rapid-acting insulin over

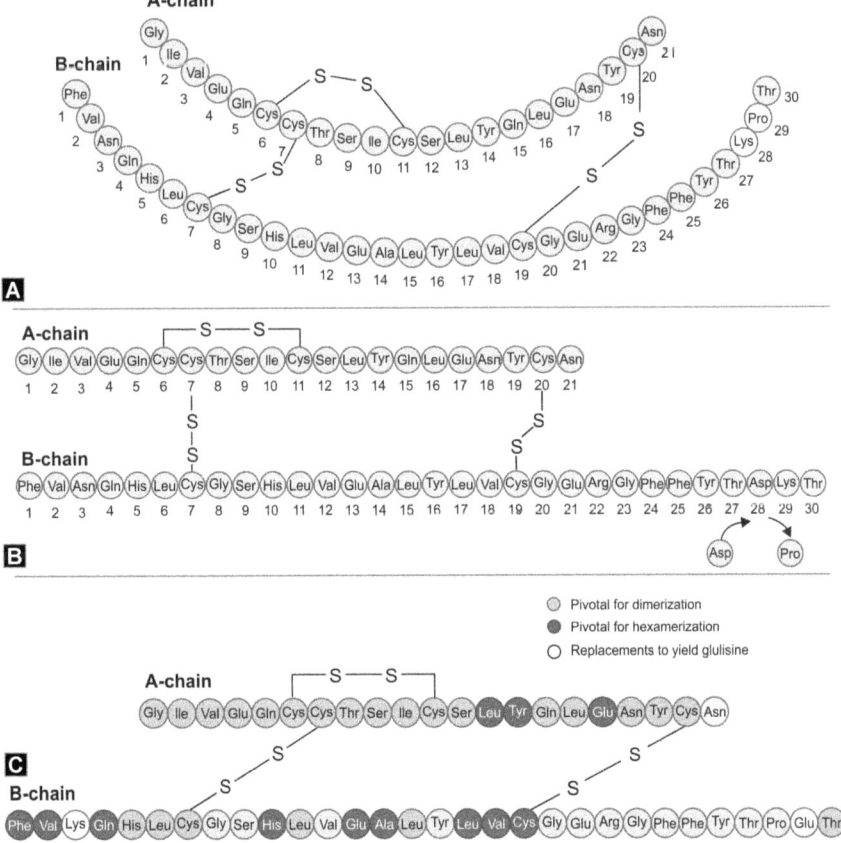

FIGS. 1A TO C: Structures of rapid-acting insulin analogs. (A) Primary structure of insulin lispro; (B) Structural formula of insulin aspart; and (C) Primary structure of insulin glulisine.
Source: White JR Insulin analogs: what are the clinical implications of structural differences? US Pharm. 2010;35(5)(Diabetes Suppl):3-7.

short-acting insulin is flexibility as regards time of administration. Short-acting insulin is relatively slowly absorbed from subcutaneous (SC) tissue and thus is required to be injected 30 minutes before meals for optimizing postprandial blood glucose levels. Unpredictable delivery of food, change of decision regarding the amount and time of food, vomiting, etc., can lead to poor postprandial control. In pursuit of minimizing above mentioned controllable variables, the patient loses his flexibility. A rapid-acting insulin is more rapidly absorbed and eliminated than short-acting insulin. Thus, postprandial blood glucose control is a bit better, and also chances of late postprandial hypoglycemia are a bit lesser than in those using rapid-acting insulin as compared to short-acting insulin. Because of quicker absorption, rapid-acting insulin is injected just 10 minutes before the meals and in case of unpredictability, even if it is administered just before food, the additional rise in postprandial blood glucose is not very significant.

Indications of rapid-acting insulin analogs are the same as those of short-acting insulin and should be preferred over them whenever postprandial blood glucose control is inadequate or there is a higher prevalence of late postprandial hypoglycemia, or the patient wants flexibility. Among those without financial constrain, prandial insulin therapy can be directly started with rapid-acting insulin.

Ultrarapid-acting Insulin (Fiasp)

In Fiasp, niacinamide, which facilitates absorption from SC tissues at a slightly faster rate than rapid-acting insulin; and an amino acid arginine, which stabilizes it, are added to aspart. It has two advantages over rapid-acting insulin. When the time or amount of food consumed or retained is unpredictable, it can be given just before, with, or up to 20 minutes after food. Comparative studies have shown that 1-hour postprandial blood glucose levels are better with Fiasp than aspart. In short, it is one step ahead of the three rapid-acting insulins. Ultrarapid-acting lispro, which has similar pharmacokinetic advantages over rapid and short-acting insulin, is not yet available in India.

Indications for ultrarapid-acting Fiasp are the same as those of rapid-acting insulin. Its advantages over rapid-acting insulin include more flexibility, better 1-hour postprandial control, and slightly lesser cost.

Intermediate-acting Insulin

Neutral protamine Hagedorn (NPH) insulin containing protamine and zinc to prolong the duration of action of insulin is the only intermediate-acting insulin available in the market. Lente insulin which had similar pharmacokinetics has been withdrawn. The onset of action of NPH insulin is 2-4 hours after administration, peak action occurs between 6 and 10 hours after administration, while an effective duration of action is for 10-16 hours. As compared to long-acting insulin, intermediate-acting insulin has the following disadvantages: (1) Shorter duration of action, thus not covering 24 hours span and (2) peak effect around 8 hours, thus higher chances of hypoglycemia around 6–10 hours after injection, particularly when the dose is increased to improve fasting blood glucose control. Neutral protamine Hagedorn insulin is still very commonly used in a day-to-day practice as a substitute for long-acting insulin because it is inexpensive as compared to long-acting insulin. The disadvantages described above can be partly overcome by administering it twice-a-day in those with severe insulin deficiency (all type 1 diabetes mellitus (T1DM) patients and those long-standing type 2 diabetes mellitus (T2DM) patients with severe β-cell failure); or at late-night (postdinner, around 10–11 PM) in once-a-day dosage in those with small to moderate insulin requirements. The idea is to maintain adequate blood and liver insulin levels from dawn to prebreakfast time. When intermediate insulin is injected before dinner, particularly in early diners such as Jains, its levels start dwindling by dawn and early morning, when counter-regulatory hormones are at their peak. The combined effect can lead to a sharp rise in blood glucose levels in the morning. If the reason behind this phenomenon is misunderstood and predinner dose of NPH insulin is increased, there is too much insulin in circulation at around 3 AM, leading to hypoglycemia at that time. This can be avoided by shifting the time of injection of intermediate-acting insulin to around 10–11 PM. This action helps to avoid reactive morning hyperglycemia by avoiding 3 AM hypoglycemia (Somogi effect). Neutral protamine Hagedorn insulin is a genetically engineered human insulin having an identical amino acid structure as native human insulin. The difference in pharmacokinetic profile between it and short-acting insulin is due to the addition of protamine and zinc in insulin suspension. The main indication for intermediate-acting insulin is for the provision of basal insulinization.

- It can be used as a solo insulin in those with some β-cell activity still intact [clinical pointers—relatively shorter duration of diabetes, glycated hemoglobin (HbA1c) 7.5–8.0% with two to three oral antidiabetic drugs (OADs) on board]. The ideal time to inject it is around 10–11 PM. Since it does not produce a sharp peak action, there is no need for the patient to take a snack after injection. In those requiring 20 units or more, it should be given in two doses, one in the morning and the second dose at 10 PM. In those on short-acting insulin for postprandial glucose control, morning doses can be given together with short-acting insulin.
- It can be used as a basal component of basal-bolus therapy. (Clinical pointers—long-standing diabetics or those with complications; and having poor glycemic control and those who have failed to reach glycemic targets with basal insulin plus OAD therapy). In such indications, short-acting insulin is coadministered with intermediate-acting insulin.
- Intermediate-acting (NPH) insulin is still in common use because of its cost advantage; it has no pharmacological advantage over long-acting insulin. Thus, among those without financial constrain, it should be replaced by long-acting insulin.

However, please note that NPH insulin is still quite commonly used in India and in advanced, rich countries such as the USA and the UK, because insurance companies in the USA and government authorities in the UK, which bear the cost of healthcare in those countries respectively, are very cost conscious. Neutral protamine Hagedorn insulin in the hands of an experienced and astute clinician is effective.

Long-acting Insulin

A normal person secretes a small amount of insulin during the basal state, In patients with severe insulin deficiency, a truly long-acting basal insulin given once-a-day is required to maintain glycemic control in the basal state, which corresponds to an entire overnight period till the breakfast, and a short period in the evening till dinner, to suppress excessive hepatic glucose production. Till the availability of long-acting insulin, NPH insulin was used to provide basal insulinization. The research and development on long-acting insulin analogs having smoother, truly round-the-clock action without significant episodes of hypoglycemia started simultaneously with that of rapid-acting analogs and we now have many long and ultralong-acting insulin analogs to provide basal insulinization. All the current long-acting insulin preparations in the market are examples of insulin analogs.

Insulin Glargine

This long-acting analog of insulin was introduced in India about two decades back, within 1 year after its international launch. Following structural changes have been incorporated in glargine to get an improved pharmacokinetic profile. (1) In position 21 in the A chain, asparagine is replaced by glycine and (2) At the end of the B chain two arginine residues are added. It is relatively "peakless" insulin with 22–24 hours of action (refer to **Fig. 2A**). Neutral protamine Hagedorn insulin does not have round-the-clock action and thus needs to be given twice-a-day to avoid wide blood glucose fluctuations. Glargine is relatively peakless and has the following advantages over intermediate-acting insulin:
- It can be taken at any time of the day as per the patient's convenience (of course it should be taken at the same time every day).
- In most of the patients, it needs to be taken only once-a-day.
- Episodes of hypoglycemia, particularly severe and nocturnal hypoglycemia, are less as compared to NPH insulin, because of its relatively flat, peakless pharmacokinetic profile.
- It is ideal insulin to be used along with OADs for tight blood glucose control in type 2 diabetics who do not respond adequately to OADs but still have some residual β-cell function. When fasting blood glucose crosses 150 mg%, in spite of taking two or three different OADs in submaximal to maximal doses, one may continue the pills and add glargine 10 units daily and gradually increase if required. It will lead to better blood glucose control.

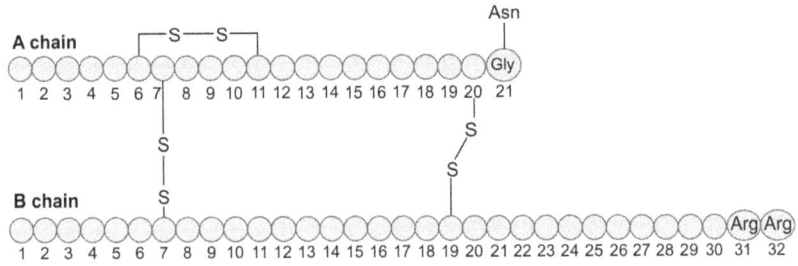

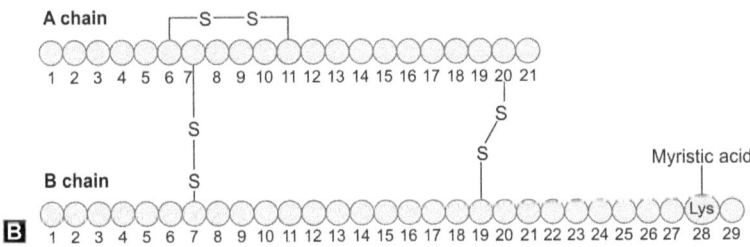

FIGS. 2A AND B: Structures of long-acting insulin analogs. (A) Primary structure of insulin glargine and (B) Primary structure of insulin detemir.
Source: White JR Insulin analogs: what are the clinical implications of structural differences? US Pharm. 2010;35(5)(Diabetes Suppl):3–7.

- It can also be used as a basal insulin component in any intensive insulin therapy, which is usually required in type 1 diabetics and severe type 2 diabetics with secondary failure to oral agents. In this plan, glargine is given once-a-day, and short- or rapid-acting insulin is separately given before each meal. A usual starting dose of glargine is 10 units once-a-day. It may be noted that glargine should not be mixed with any other insulin in the same syringe. Late-night timing (between 10 and 11 PM) is advisable because it provides some flexibility. Even on days when the patient's return to home is delayed or when he plans an evening outing, he can still come back and take insulin at the usual time so that his glycemic control is not disturbed. Evening dose is preferred to the morning dose to provide adequate hepatic insulinization in the early morning in those minority of patients in whom glargine provides therapeutic insulin levels for a couple of hours lesser than 24 hours. In such patients, if glargine is administered in morning, subtherapeutic insulin levels superadded with excessive counter-regulatory hormone levels can spoil fasting glucose levels. This is avoided by administering glargine in the evening, by preventing coincidence of tail end subtherapeutic insulin levels and peak counter-regulatory hormone levels.
- In short glargine has same indications as those of intermediate-acting insulin and when cost constrain is not an issue, glargine should be preferred.

Concentrated (U-300) Glargine

It is a glargine formulation in three times concentrated form and resultant smaller size of deposited mass in SC tissue after injection is one of the reasons leading to slower release of insulin crystals as compared to glargine 100, with which it shares exactly the same amino acid structure. As compared to conventional glargine (U-100), concentrated (U-300) form of glargine has a flatter pharmacokinetic profile and slightly longer duration of action. It is true once-a-day insulin. In some patients who have difficulty in controlling their fasting blood glucose with glargine, one may consider using glargine (300 units). As compared to glargine, hypoglycemic episodes, particularly nighttime episodes, occur at a lesser frequency.

Detemir Insulin

It was the first long-acting insulin analog to be marketed anywhere. The following structural changes have been incorporated in detemir: (1) Amino acid at position B30 has been removed and (2) myristic acid side chain has been attached to amino acid 29 in the B chain (refer to **Fig. 2B**). These changes are responsible for a long duration of action. Like glargine, detemir is a long-acting insulin analog with generally similar pharmacokinetics and indications. It has a slightly shorter duration of action than glargine. Thus, even though it works on once-a-day basis in many type 2 diabetics, some patients, particularly those having type 1 diabetes are better off with twice-a-day dosing of detemir. In fact, in European countries it is mandatory to prescribe it twice-a-day. Weight gain in patients on detemir is a bit less than those on equal doses of other insulin preparations. With the availability of 24-hour-acting peakless insulin such as glargine 300 and degludec, use of detemir has come down considerably. It is the only long-acting insulin which has category B status for use in pregnancy, thus preferred in this indication.

Degludec

This long-acting basal insulin analog was introduced in India in September 2013. It has a truly 24-hour long action span, as its biological half-life is 42 hours. The following structural changes are responsible for its long action: (1) Removal of amino acid from position 30 and (2) attachment of a fatty acid, hexadecanedioic acid through a spacer at B29 (refer to **Fig. 3**). Its other advantages over traditional long-acting insulin are (1) flexibility as regards timing of insulin injection, since it has a long biological half-life, unlike other basal insulin preparations, the patient is not likely to lose glycemic control even if he delays his insulin injection by a few hours. Thus, in case patient forgets to take an insulin injection at the scheduled time or is unable to take it due to logistic reasons, he can take it as soon as he remembers or as soon as he can take it. Subsequently, he should continue his 24-hourly schedule. At least 8 hours must elapse between two injections. This is a big plus point; (2) hypoglycemia—the frequency and severity of hypoglycemia, particularly nocturnal hypoglycemia is less with insulin degludec as compared with

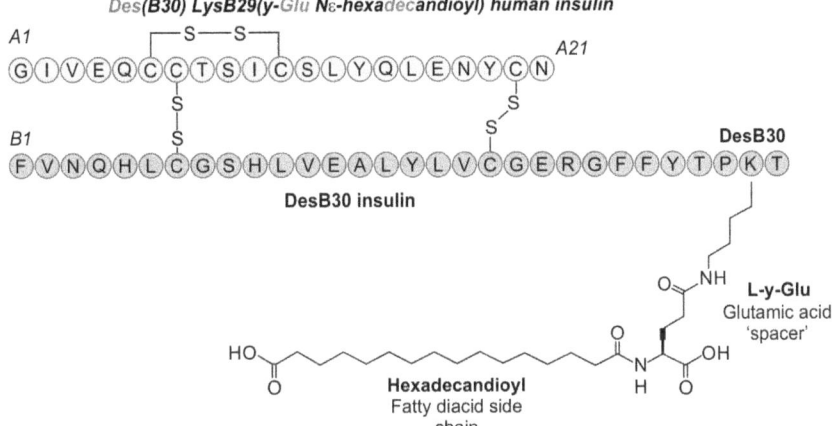

FIG. 3: Insulin degludec.
Source: Jonassen I, Havelund S, Hoeg-Jensen T, Steensgaard DB, Wahlund PO, Ribel U. Design of the novel protraction mechanism of insulin degludec, an ultra-long-acting basal insulin. 2012;29(8):2104-14.

insulin glargine. Glargine 300 nearly matches the pharmacokinetic profile of degludec and shares most of the advantages including flexibility as regards time of injection. Though far more flexible as compared to glargine and detemir, as regards time of injection, it is less flexible than degludec (3 hours extension vs. 8 hours extension).

Degludec is ideal basal insulin and can be combined with short or rapid-acting insulin preparations in basal-bolus insulin therapy for type 1 diabetic patients and some of the type 2 diabetic patients. It can also be used along with metformin or other oral antidiabetic agents in type 2 diabetic patients with some β-cell activity. However, degludec is costlier than glargine. Refer to **Table 3** for comparative pharmacokinetic profiles of all insulin preparations on the market.

In short, we have five insulin preparations for basal insulinization, namely:
1. *NPH insulin*: Most economical with many limitations.
2. *Detemir*: Pharmacokinetically better but costlier insulin was the basal insulin of choice for a short time in first decade of this century, till still better basal insulin preparations came in the market. Now gradually fading away.
3. *Glargine*: Good basal insulin but has some limitations as compared to glargine 300 and degludec, but at the same time very clear superiority over NPH insulin. Cost has come down, several generics have entered the market, thus the cost will come down further.
4. *Glargine 300 and degludec*: True 24 hours-acting peakless insulin preparations. Some advantages over glargine but the cost difference is not insignificant.

Thus, the clinician has a wide choice and should decide depending upon the individual patient's clinical needs and economic considerations

TABLE 3: Summary of insulin pharmacokinetics.

Generic name	Brand names	Time of onset of action (hours)	Time to peak action (hours)	Duration of action (hours)
Regular human	Actrapid	0.5	1.5–2.5	8
Aspart	NovoRapid	Within 0.25	0.5–1.5	4–6
Fast-acting aspart	Fiasp	Within 0.25	1	2–4
Lispro	Humalog	Within 0.25	0.5–1.5	4–6
Glulisine	Apidra	Within 0.25	0.5–1.5	4–6
Neutral protamine Hagedorn (NPH)	Insulatard	2–4	4–10	12–18
Detemir	Levemir	2–4	Flat	14–24
Glargine 100	Lantus	2–4	Flat	20–24
Glargine 300	Toujeo	6	Flat	Up to 36
Degludec	Tresiba	1	Flat	>42

Source: In: White JR (Ed). 2022-23 Guide to Medications for the Treatment of Diabetes Mellitus. Los Angeles: American Diabetes Association; 2022.

Premixed Insulin

Ready-made insulin mixtures of short-acting insulin and intermediate-acting NPH insulin are available in 25/75, 30/70, and 50/50 proportions, these are called *premixed insulin*. Mixtures of rapid-acting analogs, lispro, and aspart are also available in 30/70 (aspart) or 25/75 (lispro) and 50/50 (aspart/lispro) proportions with NPH insulin. Some patients have difficulty in mixing insulin. For such patients, these mixtures are useful. Depending upon individual needs, a particular mixture can be selected.

Pros and Cons of Premixed Insulin Preparations

One must note that the flexibility of independently altering either short-acting/rapid-acting or intermediate-acting components of insulin is lost with ready-made mixtures. When one increases or decreases the dose of such mixtures, both the components are proportionately altered. In other words, insulin mixtures are like readymade garments, they do not suit everybody (one size does not necessarily fit all). The convenience of the ready mixture comes with the limitations regarding flexibility of dosages. If a given mixture can provide both the short/rapidacting and intermediate-acting components in exact units as per the individual need, then mixtures are suitable. This is as far as the theoretical limitations of insulin mixtures; however, in real-life situations, if a patient ideally requires individual insulin preparations to be mixed manually, just cannot master the process of mixing insulin, or does not have any intention of learning the same—it is far better to prescribe ready premixed insulin if he can manage to take it. After all, theoretical limitations apart, HbA1c of 8% is far better than 10%. Many primary care physicians are also not very confident of prescribing full basal-bolus insulin therapy in their patients. Because of all these reasons, premixed insulin is very commonly prescribed in India and developing countries. For your information, Mixtard is the number one prescribed medicine in India. Its sales are more than any other medicine in India, across all categories of medicines. Premixed insulin with 30% short-acting components is used as staple premixed insulin. Those on this insulin with difficulty in achieving postprandial glucose control can be shifted to a 50/50 premixed concentration. But keep the possibility of spoiling control 7–8 hours down the line due to automatic reduction in intermediate-acting insulin concentration from 70 to 50%. Remember the famous English proverb *"You can't always have a cake and eat it too."*

Indications for Premixed Insulin

Premixed insulin preparations provide a pragmatic alternative to basal-bolus insulin therapy or basal-plus insulin therapy. In the initial period of basal alone insulin therapy failure, one can use premixed insulin once-a-day instead of separately administering NPH/long-acting insulin plus short-acting/rapid-acting insulin. It should be administered 30 minutes before (human premixed insulin), or 10 minutes before (premixed analogs) the meal responsible for the highest postprandial peak. If and when further intensification is required, premix insulin twice and occasionally thrice a day can be used as a pragmatic alternative to basal-bolus therapy. Those taking premixed insulin twice-a-day should keep a gap of at least 6 hours between the two injections (in other words, one of the two injections should be taken before dinner and the other before breakfast or lunch). Premixed analogs are costlier than premixed human insulin preparations but provide slightly better postprandial glucose control and also produce lesser late postprandial hypoglycemia episodes.

Coformulated Insulin

Coformulation of aspart with degludec is available under the trade name Ryzodeg. Differences between coformulation and premix insulin are: (1) In the former, both the components retain separate identities and their individual pharmacokinetic properties and (2) the longer-acting component in Ryzodeg is degludec, the true 24-hour-acting insulin, whereas in premixed insulin, it is NPH insulin, which is an intermediate-acting insulin. The intermediate-acting component of premixed insulin is in suspension and thus settles down in the container when not in use. In order to make uniform suspension before injection, the patient or his helper should roll the vial or pen between the palms 8–10 times in order to maintain the same proportion of two components in the injected insulin dose. This step is often bypassed either due to lack of awareness or in a hurry, this is likely to result in changed pharmacokinetics of injected insulin leading to hypoglycemia in the early postinjection period or hyperglycemia, a few hours later. Thus, three clinical benefits of coformulated insulin over premixed insulin are (1) lower chances of late postprandial hypoglycemia due to absence of "shoulder effect" or prolongation of action span of shorter-acting insulin, (2) better-fasting blood glucose control due to superiority of degludec over intermediate-acting insulin, and (3) laser day-to-day variability.

■ REAL-LIFE SITUATION

In Chapter 6, we reviewed the physiology and pathophysiology of insulin secretion and in this chapter; we went through the phrmacokinetics of various human and analog insulin formulations. We have also reviewed spectacular evolutionary improvements in the quality of insulin over the last 100 years. The fresh and young clinician would be very eager now to translate all the aforementioned information into clinical practice and start prescribing insulin based on his newly acquired information. He may take success in terms of swift glycemic control for granted.

Now, before going into the clinical aspects of insulin therapy let me warn young clinicians that things are not always hunky-dory. Though you are using human insulin which has exactly the same amino acid structure as that of native insulin and same purity, it is delivered in very unnatural way. In the normal, nondiabetic person, insulin is synthesized in the pancreas and released directly into the portal circulation, whereas when a patient with diabetes is prescribed insulin, he has no other alternative but to inject it in SC tissue from where it enters the systemic circulation and only a small portion of injected insulin reaches portal circulation after first passing through the entire systemic circulation. Thus, it results in excess of insulin at sites where it is not required and relative deficiency of insulin in portal circulation. In addition, the normal pancreas secrets insulin continuously for 24 hours while in diabetic patients it is usually injected one to three times daily. In normal persons, insulin release is automatically controlled by prevalent blood glucose. As the blood glucose starts falling, insulin release is inhibited and glucagon release is stimulated, when the blood glucose starts rising, as in postprandial period, insulin release is stimulated while glucagon release is inhibited. Insulin administered externally in SC tissue is not under biofeedback-related automatic control. In addition, multiple factors can alter the rate of absorption of subcutaneously administered insulin in circulation. After exercise, massage of the part of the body where insulin is injected, or after a hot bath, insulin will be absorbed faster, while if injected in a cold atmosphere, it will be absorbed slower. If by mistake, it is injected intramuscularly, it will be absorbed faster. This can occasionally happen with the wrong injection technique in extremely thin people. Insulin is absorbed faster from abdominal SC tissue as compared to from thigh, buttock and arms. Not keeping an appropriate time gap between the injection of short-acting insulin and food intake can also alter the outcome. Patient noncompliance or partial compliance, inadequate knowledge of clinician as regards choosing right insulin in right dose and judicious dosage adjustment are some of the additional factors responsible for inadequate glycemic control in spite of insulin, often in large dosage, in some of the patients. When such a mismatch occurs, resultant hypoglycemia or hyperglycemia disturbs the patient and reduces his compliance further while it disturbs the confidence of an inexperienced clinician. Be rest assured that, though things can go wrong, they do not go wrong in everybody, many patients do exceptionally well and others gradually improve when the cause of inadequate control is systematically analyzed and remedial actions taken. After all, in almost all the clinical trials, including those in real world set ups, insulin has invariably given better results than any noninsulin antidiabetic agent. Furthermore, while all other antidiabetic agents have some contraindications, insulin has none.

▪ WHICH PATIENTS NEED INSULIN?

Patients with type 1 diabetes should be put on insulin immediately after the diagnosis as their life is dependent on it and they would develop diabetic ketoacidosis leading to coma, if insulin is withheld.

▪ GENERAL PRINCIPLES OF INSULIN ADMINISTRATION IN THE MANAGEMENT OF TYPE 1 DIABETES MELLITUS

Types 1 diabetes mellitus is associated with total destruction of β-cells and thus, total absence of endogenous insulin synthesis. As insulin plays a major physiological role in the metabolism of carbohydrates as well as proteins and fats, exogenous insulin administration is mandatory for survival of patients with type 1 diabetes. In an environment devoid of insulin, all noninsulin antidiabetic agents except sodium-glucose cotransporter-2 inhibitors (SGLT-2Is) and alpha-glucosidase inhibitors (AGIs) are ineffective, or minimally effective as adjuncts in those with additional insulin resistance (metformin and pioglitazone). SGLT-2Is and AGIs, though effective, have limited efficacy in bringing down HbA1c anywhere near the goal in such a situation. Thus, exogenously administered insulin has to do all the bull work of establishing glycemic control. As they have severe insulin deficiency, type 1 diabetic patients require a combination of basal and bolus insulin to maintain round-the-clock tissue insulinization. Basal insulin maintains glycemic control by preventing overproduction of glucose in lever through a check on neoglucogenesis and glycogenolysis in liver, while prandial insulin administered before major meals checks excessive rise of blood glucose levels in postprandial period. Thus, in a majority of type 1 diabetic patients, basal-bolus insulin therapy with administration of once or twice daily long-acting or intermediate-acting insulin respectively, along with prandial insulin before major meals, is the mainstay of antidiabetic therapy. Due to total absence of endogenous insulin, less intensive insulin therapies such a basal only or prandial only therapy is unlikely to be successful in reaching glycemic targets, due to inadequate control on fasting/premeal glucose control with bolus only therapies and poor fasting blood glucose control with prandial only therapies. Furthermore, total insulin dose required per day is higher as compared that required by patients having type 2 diabetes. At initiation, the recommended dose per day is 0.6 U/kg of body weight.

Primary care clinicians have much larger experience of using insulin in type 2 diabetic patients, in whom, depending upon the individual patient's current β-cell functional status, varying amount of endogenous insulin is available which works along with externally administered insulin. Coadministration of sulfonylureas (SUs), meglitinides, glucagon-like peptide-1 receptor agonists (GLP-1 RAs), and dipeptidyl peptidase-4 inhibitors (DPP-4Is) can increase endogenous insulin secretion to varying extent, depending upon individual patient's β-cell functional capacity; and insulin sensitizers can increase the sensitivity of tissues to externally administered and endogenously secreted insulin. Sodium-glucose cotransporter-2 inhibitors and AGIs have insulin-independent mechanisms of action through which they reduce HbA1c to a limited extent in any diabetic patient irrespective of the functional capacity of their β-cells. Thus, in these patients, less intensive insulin therapies such as basal-only insulin often work very well, till the time their β-cells have some functional capacity. Type 1 diabetics do not have any capacity to secrete insulin. Thus, agents working through β-cell stimulation and sensitization of tissues to insulin do not work in type 1 diabetes and HbA1c reduction through insulin independent action is too small to bring HbA1c to the goal. Thus, type 1 diabetics require more intensive insulin therapy such as basal-bolus insulin therapy, which includes basal insulin providing round-the-clock tissue insulinization, and prandial insulin to cover all major meals, right from the initiation stage.

In short primary care physicians should remember that need for insulin and extent of intensification of insulin cannot be solely decided by prevalent glycemic control. Type of diabetes, age of the patient, duration of diabetes, response to current therapy, associated comorbidities and complications, degree of insulin resistance, etc.; all these factors require consideration while making decisions about antidiabetic treatment. A recently diagnosed 40-year-old asymptomatic patient with type 2 diabetes quickly responds to OADs, even if his baseline glycemic control is very poor, while true type 1 diabetic patient will not have good HbA1c values even if his fasting blood glucose is reasonably controlled with best basal insulin on the board.

■ TEMPORARY REMISSION IN TYPE 1 DIABETES MELLITUS

Some type 1 diabetic patients go into temporary remission within days or weeks after starting insulin therapy. This is due to swift reestablishment of glycemic control leading to control of glucotoxicity and lipotoxicity related potentially reversible depression of small number of still viable β-cells. During the remission state, which lasts for up to few weeks to months, glycemic control can be obtained with less intensive and simpler insulin regimens, or even without insulin in some cases, but after some weeks, when autoimmune destruction of β-cells is complete; these patients usually require full basal-bolus insulin therapy. Such patients require close monitoring of their glycemic status through structured self-monitoring program so that recurrent hypoglycemic episodes in the initial period of remission and subsequent prolonged hyperglycemia during the period when patients are coming out of remission can be minimized.

■ OVERLAPPING FEATURES BETWEEN TYPE 1 DIABETES MELLITUS AND TYPE 2 DIABETES MELLITUS IN ADOLESCENTS AND YOUNG ADULTS

Type 2 diabetes mellitus in adolescents and young adults is quite common nowadays. These patients are usually obese, have other features of insulin resistance, such as acanthosis nigricans, raised triglyceride level in blood, and hypertension. Thus, in those with very high blood glucose levels at presentation, they are likely to be misdiagnosed as type 1 diabetes, which used to be overwhelmingly predominant subtype of diabetes at that age group till two decades ago. In such severely symptomatic patients with very high blood glucose, it is prudent to start the treatment with insulin, even if one picks up the clues suggesting a strong possibility of type 2 diabetes. Absent glutamic acid decarboxylase (GAD) and islet cell antibodies and rapid need for de intensification of insulin therapy are indirect proofs of patient having type 2 diabetes. These patients can be gradually shifted to metformin.

Please use the information given in the last two paragraphs to differentiate between type 1 diabetes in "honeymoon period" masquerading as type 2 diabetes and severe type 2 diabetes in obese insulin resistant young adults masquerading as type 1 diabetes and use appropriate insulin therapy as per the individual patient's need.

Insulin in Type 2 Diabetes Mellitus

About 95–96% of diabetics in our country have T2DM. At any given point of time, around 60% of them can be controlled on diet and OAD's. However, in the following circumstances, insulin should be used:
- During severe stressful situations, e.g., septicemia, tuberculosis, other severe infections, myocardial infarction, etc. During such situations, there is an increase in counter-regulatory hormone secretion in response to stressful situations. Under such conditions, lifestyle changes and OADs are not sufficient to establish and maintain glycemic control.
- During perioperative period in patients undergoing major surgery
- During pregnancy and lactation
- In those patients in whom the highest dosage of OADs from two/three different groups fails to bring down blood glucose levels to normal
- When OADs are contraindicated (e.g., severe hepatic and renal failure)
- When patients present with very high-glucose levels [fasting blood sugar (FBS) > 300 mg%, postprandial blood sugar (PPBS) > 400 mg%, and HbA1c > 10.5%] associated with severe symptoms such as polyuria, polydipsia and weight loss.

■ INITIATION OF INSULIN TREATMENT

Acutely ill patients requiring changeover to insulin, or all newly diagnosed T1DM patients requiring insulin, should be preferably admitted for a few days for initiation, dosage adjustment, and training regarding insulin injection techniques, method of monitoring and also for training regarding prevention/detection and self-treatment of hypoglycemia. The opportunity should also be utilized for patient education program on various other aspects of diabetes.

Now, let us see how to handle insulin initiation in outpatient practice. Kindly note that the information given below is predominantly aimed at management of type 2 diabetes with insulin; however, the general principles of management of type 2 and type 1 diabetes with insulin are the same. Insulin dosage planning and glycemic monitoring in long-standing type 2 diabetics with end stage β-cell failure is very similar to the management of type 1 diabetic. Most of the type 1 patients with diabetes will straightaway start with full-fledged basal-bolus insulin therapy, while many patients with type 2 diabetes will start with basal-only insulin on the top of OADs. Many of these patients will require intensification to basal-plus insulin therapy and subsequently to basal-bolus insulin therapy as their β-cell function gradually deteriorates further due to progressive nature of the disease. Some of these patients with recent worsening of glycemic control due to temporary insulin resistance caused by associated complications such as severe infections, or due to temporary need of steroids to check associated conditions, may need deintensification of insulin therapy, e.g., from basal-plus to basal only or from basal-bolus to basal-plus insulin therapy.

Now, let us first understand the action spans of different insulin formulations. The prebreakfast, short-acting and rapid-acting insulin control blood glucose rise following breakfast and to some extent following lunch, while intermediate-acting insulin controls blood glucose levels mainly from afternoon period up to dinner time when injected in morning and overnight period when injected in evening. In other words, when the effect of short/rapid-acting insulin starts wearing off; intermediate-acting insulin takes over. Similarly, predinner short/rapid-acting insulin controls blood glucose rise following dinner, while predinner intermediate-acting insulin takes care of blood glucose control during the late-night and early morning period up to breakfast time. Long-acting insulin provides basal needs for 24 hours.

Insulin Initiation

The starting dose depends on several factors, including blood glucose level, associated complications and infections, capacity of β-cells to synthesize and release insulin (about 50% of the β-cells are functional at the time of onset of T2DM and as time passes, the percentage of the β-cells which are functional, gradually reduces), insulin resistance (judged by weight of the patient and other signs), etc. Usual starting dose 0.2 U/kg body weight/24 hours. Obese patients are insulin resistant and usually require a higher starting dose.

In a day-to-day practice, even among those patients consulting for the first time, a clinician sees patients at different stages of their journey with diabetes with varying degree of glycemic control and varying capacity of β-cells. Thus, each patient's insulin requirements at the time of initiation are different. Some are suitable for a simple basal-alone initiation plan. Some with very poor glycemic control and underlying complications will need a full-fledged basal-bolus therapy at the time of insulin initiation itself, while others may need a moderately intensified plan such at basal-plus insulin therapy. In those with predominantly fasting hyperglycemia, and in whom insulin is being introduced fairly early and at appropriate time, entire daily dose can be given at bedtime in the form of intermediate or long-acting insulin (basal-alone insulin therapy). In others with pointers suggesting more severe β-cell deficiency and/or associated significant insulin resistance, such as more severe hyperglycemia, long duration of diabetes, associated severe infections, other stressful conditions, and obesity, one needs to start with higher dose, such as 0.3–0.4 kg/body weight/24 hours. Those requiring higher dosages and more intensified insulin initiation will need a combination of basal and bolus insulin. In these patients, out of total number of units calculated, half the number of units are given as short-acting or rapid-acting insulin and the remaining as intermediate-acting insulin or long-acting insulin.

INSULIN REGIMENS IN TYPE 2 DIABETES MELLITUS

Basal-alone Regimen

Ambulatory patients who have diabetes for a relatively short period, but not responding to two to three oral agents and have HbA1c < 8.5% and FBS and PPBS values not more than 150–160 and 220–250 respectively can respond to once-a-day intermediate-acting or long-acting insulin plus OADs because the aforementioned clinical pointers indicate that there are still a few months or years left before they reach severe β-cell failure state. The decision between intermediate or long-acting insulin will depend upon the affordability. Long-acting insulin has very clear advantages over intermediate insulin. The starting dose is usually 10 units once-a-day or 0.2 U/kg body weight. Intermediate-acting insulin is given around 10 PM, while true long-acting insulin can be given at any time of the day, but at the same time every day (glargine 100/detemir). If degludec or glargine 300 is used as a long-acting insulin, some leniency as regards timing is allowed as an exception. The reason for giving intermediate-acting insulin at late-night is to ensure that during the "Dawn phenomenon" time (4–10 AM), plasma concentration of intermediate-acting insulin is at its peak and not on a downward slope. By adopting this strategy, one can minimize the morning hyperglycemic spurt, which is difficult to control in some patients. Shifting injection time from predinner to late-night leads to shifting the peak plasma level of intermediate-acting insulin from predawn to dawn and early morning and blunting of early morning hyperglycemia.

Insulin Dose Adjustments

In those on basal-alone insulin, fasting blood glucose is monitored for adjustment of insulin dosage. Advice the patient to estimate it daily and every third or fourth day calculate the mean blood glucose and adjust the insulin dosage as per **Table 4**. It has been observed that self-adjustment of insulin dosage leads to increased patient involvement, boosts his self-confidence and is associated with better outcomes as compared to adjustments made by the treating doctor. In those with impaired cognitive functions, the treating doctor has to take over this aspect directly or through medical or trained nursing staff and patient's relatives or caretakers.

If patients require >20 units of intermediate-acting insulin, it should be divided into two equal doses and the additional dose should be given in the morning and they should monitor predinner blood glucose to adjust the morning dose of insulin and use **Table 4** to adjust the morning dose of intermediate-acting insulin in similar way. It is prudent to first tackle fasting blood glucose and subsequently adjust the morning insulin dose as per predinner blood glucose levels. Estimate HbA1c every three months. If not at goal, do postprandial blood glucose estimations at different times to find out the pattern, or do continuous glucose monitoring (CGM), and intensify insulin therapy by adding 2–4 units of short-acting insulin before the meal responsible for the highest postprandial blood glucose. Thus, basal-only insulin is intensified to the next level of basal-plus insulin therapy. If the patient is on long-acting insulin for basal insulinization, it should be given in single dose till the dose exceeds 0.5 units/kg of body weight. At that stage, if FBS or HbA1c is not at the goal, do multiple blood glucose monitoring or CGM and intensify insulin therapy to basal-plus therapy.

Pitfall of the Traditional Method of Administering Intermediate-acting Insulin before Dinner

This is more commonly recognized in early diners. If intermediate insulin is injected at 7 PM, the time at which its plasma level starts to dwindle exactly coincides with the time at which the counter-regulatory hormones (growth hormone, cortisol, glucagon, and epinephrine) start rising in plasma.
- *Advantages of basal-alone insulin regimen*: It is undoubtedly the simplest insulin regimen and, the, easiest way to introduce insulin therapy in reluctant patients.

TABLE 4: Dose adjustment in basal-alone insulin regimen.	
Fasting blood glucose in mg%	Insulin dose adjustment
<80	–2 units
80–125	Continue current units
126–160	+2 units
>160	+4 units

- *Disadvantages of basal-alone insulin regimen*: It is likely to work only in those patients who still have some ability to secrete their own insulin and are not near or at the end stage of β-cell failure. Type 2 diabetes mellitus being a progressive disease, basal-alone insulin is likely to work for a limited time. As the β-cell deficiency advances, it will not be possible to control postprandial blood glucose levels with basal insulin alone approach.

The subtle differences between the insulin initiation guidelines issued by associations from advanced countries and those from developing countries and the reasons for apparent differences:
- The guidelines from western countries very strongly recommend basal insulin alone as the preferred way to initiate insulin; some of them do not even make a passing remark or a footnote remark about the availability of other methods, such as premixed insulin for initiating insulin therapy. The western guidelines are meant for their own people with diabetes. The diabetic patients in the west do not have strong insulin phobia, they accept insulin therapy more easily and earlier, unlike in developing countries such as ours, where, on an average, insulin is started 7–9 years later and at a time when type 2 diabetes has progressed to near end stage β-cell failure. The basal only approach works well in the west because insulin is initiated at appropriate time, when β-cells still have some ability to produce their own insulin, which though inadequate to maintain glycemic control solely on its own, works well in combination with basal insulin and helps to simplify insulin therapy. Basal insulin alone approach fails in the majority of Indian patients because at a stage when it is usually started, there is hardly any endogenous insulin secretion, and such patients do not have a capacity to produce extra insulin on demand following food ingestion and thus require externally administered prandial insulin in addition to basal insulin. The guidelines, such as those issued by Research Society for study of diabetes in India (RSSDI), International Diabetes Federation (IDF), which addresses the global population of people with diabetes, and many developing countries, give equal importance to premixed insulin and coformulated insulin and advice the doctors to choose insulin initiation method as per the need of individual patient. Refer to **Flowchart 1** for Indian guidelines for initiation of insulin therapy in T2DM and refer to **Figure 4** for stepwise intensification of insulin therapy.

However, it must be noted that timely insulin initiation is the need of the day to consistently maintain good glycemic control and avoid complications of diabetes and in order to achieve this aim, healthcare providers should try their best to make patients understand this point and accept insulin as soon as it is necessary for maintaining optimal glycemic control. When initiated at an appropriate time, basal alone insulin therapy is undoubtedly the most appropriate, simplest and most acceptable insulin therapy and, with the availability of true long-acting insulin analogs and patient friendly

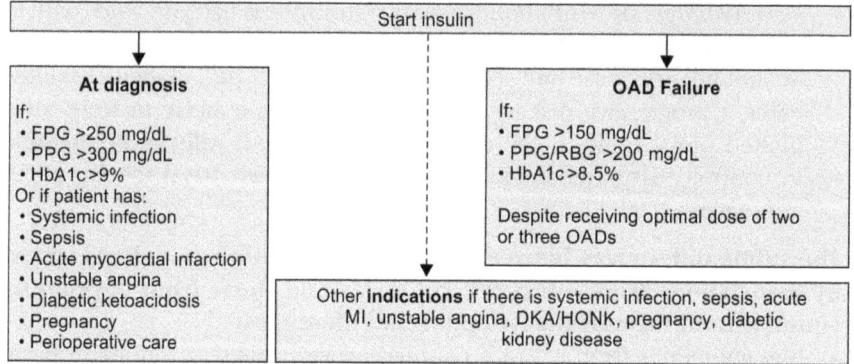

FLOWCHART 1: Indian guidelines—timely insulin initiation.
(DKA: diabetic ketoacidosis; FPG: fasting plasma glucose; HONK: hyperosmolar nonketotic coma; MI: myocardial infarction; OAD: oral antidiabetic drug; PPG: postprandial plasma glucose; RBS: random blood sugar)

Source: Indian National Consensus Group: National Guidelines on Initiation and Intensification of Insulin Therapy with Premixed Insulin Analogs. http://www.apiindia.org/contentmu2013.html

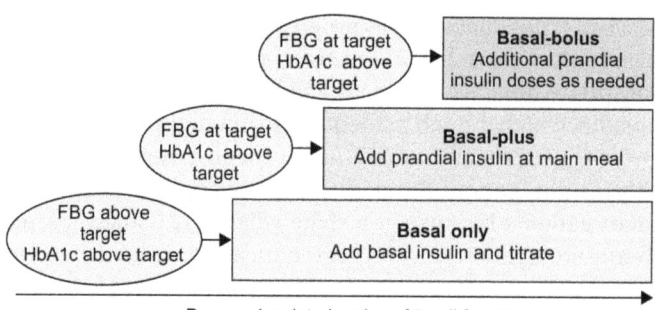

FIG. 4: Stepwise intensification of insulin treatment is required as diabetes progresses.
Source: Raccah D, Bretzel RG, Owens D, Riddle M. When basal insulin therapy in type 2 diabetes mellitus is not enough—what next? Diabtes Metab Res Rev. 2007;23(4):257-64.

injection devices, it has become even more simpler and more acceptable to the patients. If, in spite of the health care providers efforts, the opportunity to introduce basal alone insulin therapy is missed, as it is commonly occurring in present day India, one should select one of the alternative approaches, such as basal-plus, basal-bolus, and premixed insulin therapy.

When to Intensify Insulin Therapy?

In following situations, one needs to intensify the insulin regimen from basal insulin as depicted in **Flowchart 2**.

- If fasting blood glucose is above the target range in spite of administering basal insulin in the dose of 0.5 U/kg of body weight.
- If HbA1c is not lowered to the target range in spite of fasting blood glucose being in the target range.

CHAPTER 7: Insulin in the Management of Diabetes

- If one or more of postprandial blood glucose values are persistently above their target range.

Basal-plus Regimen

Those already on once-a-day basal insulin and having reasonable fasting glucose control but if HbA1c is not at the goal, it means one or more of the postprandial peaks need to be lowered. Advice the patient to estimate all the three postprandial blood glucose levels at home with a glucometer and find out the meal, which is followed by highest postprandial blood glucose level. Administer 2-4 units of short-acting insulin 30 minutes before, or rapid-acting insulin 10 minutes before the meal responsible for the highest postprandial blood glucose level. This is known as the *basal-plus 1* approach. If HbA1c is still not at the goal after tackling one postprandial peak, find out which postprandial peak is higher among the remaining two postprandial levels and if required add prandial insulin to cover that peak. This is called the *basal-plus 2* approach. If even after this regimen, HbA1c evades the goal, start full basal-bolus insulin regimen, for example, in patients on basal-plus 2 regimen with bolus insulin before breakfast and dinner, if postbreakfast blood glucose is at goal but postlunch blood glucose level is not coming down or an increase in prebreakfast short-acting insulin leads to prelunch hypoglycemia, then instead of increasing prebreakfast short-acting insulin, add a short-acting insulin before lunch.

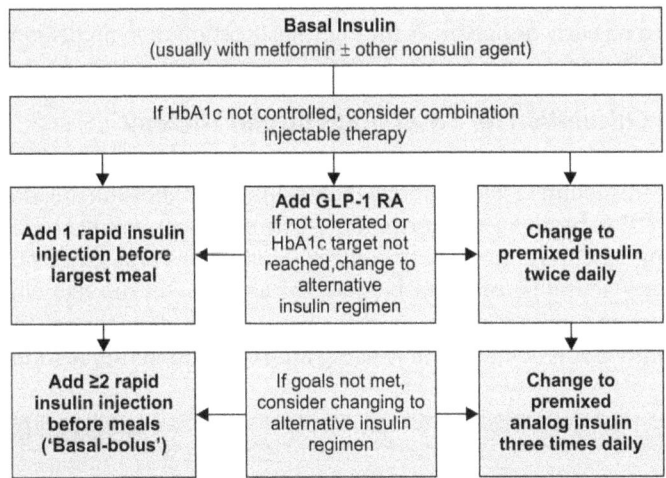

FLOWCHART 2: Intensification of insulin therapy.
(HbA1c: glycated hemoglobin; GLP-1 RA: glucagon-like peptide-1 receptor agonist)

Note: A combination of GLP-1 RA and insulin offers advantages such as neutralization of insulin induced weight gain; and reduction in incidence and severity of hypoglycemia. Furthermore, if oral semaglutide is used, or if fixed-dose combination of GLP-1 RA and insulin is used, the number of pricks can be reduced. However, both the options are extremely costly for the Indian patients spending out of their own pocket. Furthermore, fixed dose combinations of insulin with GPL-1 RA have their own limitations.

Insulin Dose Adjustments

Follow the aforementioned method for adjusting basal insulin dosage, subsequently monitor postprandial glucose corresponding to premeal insulin administration and adjust insulin dosage as per **Table 5**.

In those on basal-plus 2 prandial insulin regimen, tackle one prandial insulin dosage at a time. Estimate HbA1c every three months. If not at goal, do more frequent blood glucose estimations at different times to find out the pattern, or do CGM and intensify insulin therapy, accordingly. In short, basal-plus approach is a stop-gap approach to keep insulin therapy as simple as possible and as long as possible. (Two pricks a day are better than three and three pricks are better than full basal-bolus therapy.)

Basal-bolus Regimen

Patients already on basal-plus 2 therapy but not at glycemic goals should be intensified to basal-bolus insulin therapy. Very long standing diabetics on multiple OADs, but nowhere near glycemic targets are the candidates for basal-bolus regimen at the insulin initiation time itself. Many of these patients have significant insulin resistance due to underlying factors, such as obesity and severe infections. Those with severe hyperglycemia, osmotic symptoms, and significant weight loss at the time of diagnosis of diabetes are the candidates for basal-bolus therapy. In many of these patients, swift control of hyperglycemia with basal-bolus insulin therapy leads to rapid reversal of deleterious effects of glucotoxicity and lipotoxicity on β-cells and significant improvement in β-cell function and also reduction in insulin resistance, leading to an early opportunity for deintensification or even discontinuation of insulin therapy.

Dosage Calculation for Basal-bolus Insulin Therapy

The usual starting total daily dose (TDD) is 0.3–0.4 U/kg body weight. Obese patients are insulin resistant and usually require a higher starting dose. About 50% of TDD to be given as intermediate-acting or long-acting insulin and the remaining 50% to be divided into three equal doses and given before each meal. Long-acting insulin can be given at any time of the day while short-acting or rapid-acting insulin is given before each major meal. If, from an affordability point of view, one is using intermediate-acting insulin, one can

TABLE 5: Dose adjustment in basal-plus insulin regimen.	
Postprandial blood glucose in mg%	Prandial insulin dose adjustment
<125	–2
126–160	Continue current dose
161–200	+2
>200	+4

start with a full dose (50% of TDD) at 10 PM and subsequently split it into two doses if the TDD of intermediate-acting insulin exceeds 20 units. In such a case scenario, the additional dose is given before breakfast and can be mixed with morning's short-acting insulin. Rapid-acting insulin has an edge over short-acting insulin and should be preferred particularly in those who have difficulty in achieving postprandial glycemic control with short-acting insulin. The cost difference between short-acting and rapid-acting insulin is not insignificant.

Patients on basal-bolus insulin therapy require a more intense self-monitoring schedule. Initially, three times daily premeal blood glucose measurement is advised. Once premeal blood glucose levels are controlled, prelunch and predinner time monitoring should be replaced by monitoring of postlunch and postdinner blood glucose levels to adjust prelunch and predinner doses of short-acting insulin. To adjust the dose of prebreakfast short-acting insulin; use the prelunch blood glucose values. Once postprandial blood glucose levels are controlled, one can shift to estimation of three premeal blood glucose levels alternating with estimation of fasting, postlunch and postdinner blood glucose levels. Depending upon several factors, such as the patient's and family member's involvement, blood glucose control, clinical settings including associated conditions, affordability, etc., the monitoring schedules is modified in a pragmatic manner.

Dose Adjustment in Basal-bolus Insulin Regimen

Tackle one specific period's blood glucose at a time, starting with fasting blood glucose. **Table 5** provides information on dosage titration for fixing postprandial blood glucose level. In patients put on intermediate-acting insulin, turn your attention to predinner blood glucose level after fixing the fasting blood glucose level. If the predinner blood glucose level is above the target set for premeal blood glucose level, one has options of either adding 4–6 units of intermediate-acting insulin before breakfast or increase the dose of prebreakfast intermediate-acting insulin, if already on it, (in patients opting for syringes for insulin delivery, it can be mixed with prebreakfast or prelunch short-acting insulin to reduce the number of pricks); or increase prelunch short-acting insulin. If the increase in prelunch prandial insulin dose leads to evening time hypoglycemia, cover evening snack with 2 units of prandial insulin instead of increasing prelunch dose. In a day-to-day practice, one rarely has to resort to this step, particularly in type 2 diabetes patients. For adjusting predinner blood glucose levels, refer to **Table 4**; used for adjusting the fasting blood glucose levels. Patients on true long-acting insulin do not require a second dose and one can proceed to control of postprandial blood glucose levels directly after fixing the fasting blood glucose level. Focus your attention on postmeal values, one at a time, starting with the postmeal glucose with the highest value. **Table 5** provides information on the dosage titration for control of postprandial blood glucose values.

Handle one insulin at a time, starting with intermediate-acting or long-acting predinner insulin.
- Do not increase the dosage by >4 units at a time, unless blood glucose is extremely high or low.
- Do not increase the dosage more frequently than every third day. Before increasing the dosage, verify other variants such as missing previous insulin dose, eating an unusually large meal, etc.

Some Examples of Intensified Insulin Regimens

Figure 5 depict moderately intensified twice-daily basal-bolus therapy with NPH, along with short-acting insulin given before breakfast and dinner in two shots if syringe is used or four shots if pens are used.

Advantages: Low cost and relatively simple regimen.

Figure 6 depicts twice-a-day moderately intensified basal-bolus therapy with NPH insulin along with a rapid-acting analog. This regimen is used in those with difficulty in reaching postbreakfast or postdinner glycemic goals with aforementioned regimen.

Figures 7A and B depicts basal-bolus insulin therapy in which evening NPH insulin is shifted from before dinner time to bedtime, while retaining predinner time for evening rapid-acting insulin (**Fig. 7A** or short-acting insulin, **Fig. 7B** respectively). This strategy is employed when in pursuit of controlling fasting blood glucose leads to early morning hypoglycemia and prebreakfast hyperglycemia (Somogyi effect).

Figures 8A and B depict more intensified insulin therapy with three short/rapid-acting insulin given before each meal, and intermediate-acting insulin before breakfast along with short/rapid-acting insulin and a second

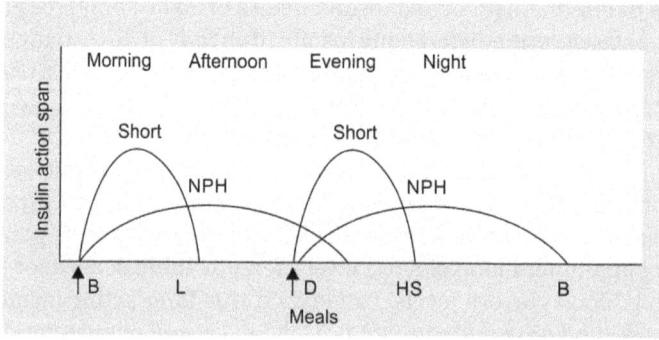

FIG. 5: Twice daily insulin regimen with short-acting and intermediate-acting insulin before breakfast and dinner.
(B: breakfast; D: dinner; HS: bedtime; L: Lunch; NPH: neutral protamine Hagedorn)

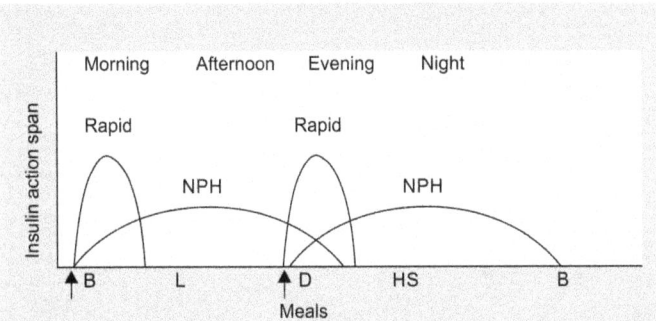

FIG. 6: Twice daily insulin regimen with rapid-acting and intermediate-acting insulin after breakfast and dinner.

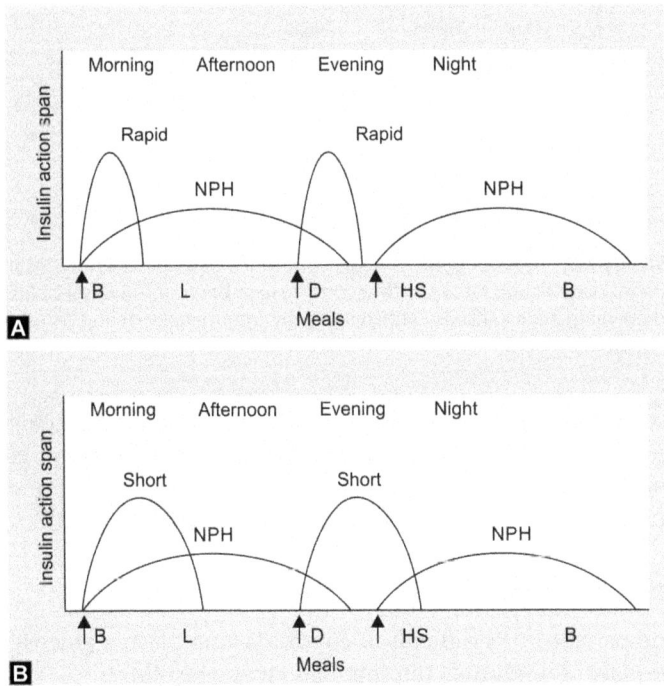

FIGS. 7A AND B: (A) Thrice daily insulin regime with bedtime NPH insulin and rapid-acting insulin. (B) Thrice daily insulin regime with bedtime NPH insulin and short-acting insulin.

dose of intermediate-acting insulin given at bedtime separately. This plan is used in patients having high post-lunch blood glucose and thus high HbA1c while on aforementioned insulin plans, which do not provide prelunch short/rapid-acting insulin.

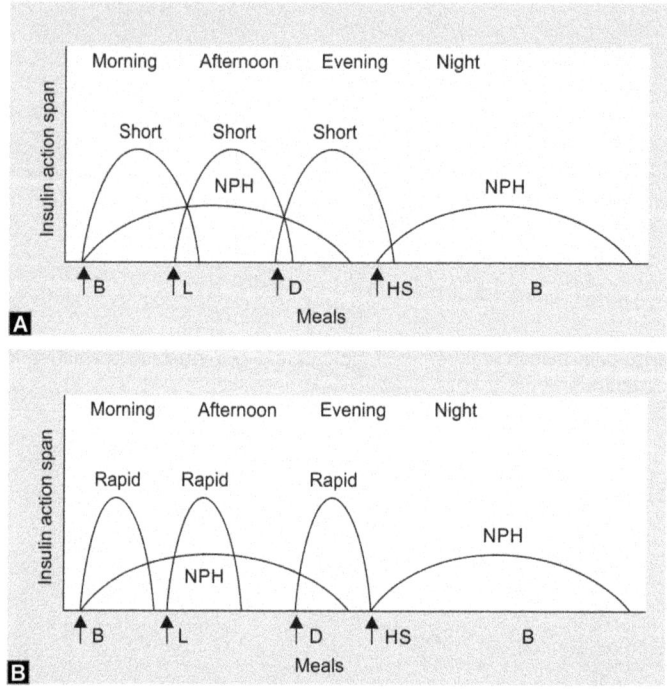

FIGS. 8A AND B: (A) Basal-bolus therapy with thrice daily short-acting insulin with twice daily intermediate-acting insulin with second dose at bedtime. (B) Basal-bolus therapy with thrice daily rapid-acting insulin with twice daily intermediate-acting insulin with second dose at bedtime.

In affording patients, therapy can be simplified by replacing two doses of intermediate-acting insulin by long-acting insulin (glargine, glargine 300, and degludec) given at bedtime. This strategy will give better-fasting and day time in between meals blood glucose control **(Figs. 9A and B)**.

■ TROUBLESHOOTING

In some patients, it is difficult to control fasting plasma glucose in spite of high dosages of predinner, intermediate-acting insulin.

Under such circumstances, giving intermediate-acting insulin at around 10–11 PM will serve the purpose. If the patient is also taking short-acting insulin before dinner, either it should be given separately before dinner, or in T2DM patients, an attempt could be made to replace it by a short-acting meglitinide such as repaglinide, DPP-4Is, and AGI. If such an attempt is successful, it will reduce the insulin injection burden. Increasing its dosage and persisting with predinner time may lead to late-night or early morning hypoglycemia with rebound hyperglycemia during the prebreakfast hours. This hyperglycemia is liable to be wrongly interpreted, resulting in further increase in predinner intermediate-acting insulin dosage.

CHAPTER 7: Insulin in the Management of Diabetes

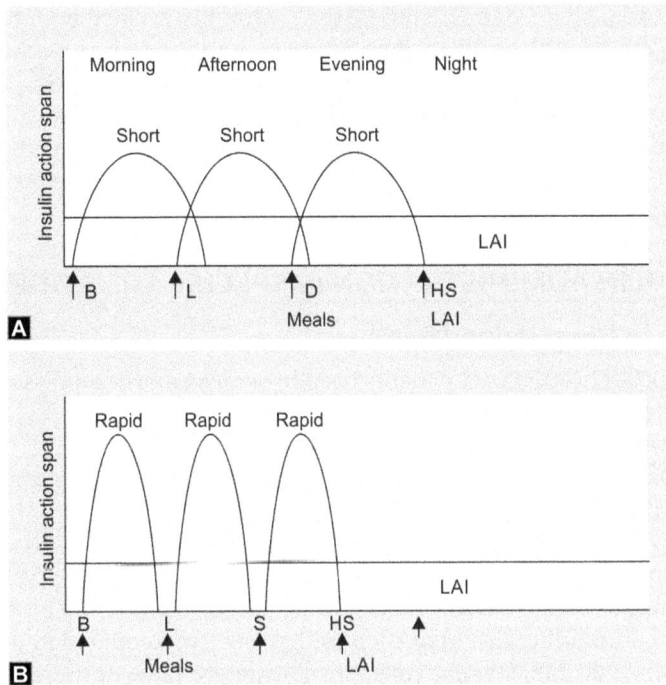

FIGS. 9A AND B: (A) Basal-bolus therapy with long-acting insulin at bedtime in combination with pre-meal short-acting insulin thrice daily. (B) Basal-bolus therapy with long-acting insulin in combination with pre-meal rapid-acting insulin thrice daily.
(LAI: long-acting insulin)

Another approach in such a situation (i.e., high fasting blood glucose in spite of 16 units of intermediate-acting insulin in the evening) is to do random blood glucose around 3 AM (by asking the patient or his relatives to do it at home with glucometer). If it is >150 mg%, increase the intermediate-acting insulin, but if it is 70 mg% or lower, reduce the intermediate-acting insulin, and you would have better control of fasting blood glucose in spite of reducing the insulin. Replacing NPH insulin with one of the peak less analogs is an excellent but expensive alternative.

What to do about OADs when Initiating or Intensifying Insulin Regimen?

If there are no contraindications to use of metformin, DPP-4Is, SGLT-2Is, and AGIs continue them along with insulin.

Long-acting SUs to be avoided and modern SU's can be continued, usually in reduced dosages. In western countries SUs are used with basal-only insulin but avoided in basal-bolus therapy, the reason being overlapping actions of externally administered insulin and endogenous insulin secreted in response to SUs. In some countries, coprescription of insulin and pioglitazone is avoided, the reason being since both can retain sodium, chances of cardiac failure are higher and incipient cardiac failure can be missed even by an experienced clinician. In patients having very poor glycemic control in spite of a large dose of insulin, some diabetologists in India are using this combination while very carefully monitoring the patient. Under such situations, insulin sensitizing action of pioglitazone occasionally works wonders.

INSULIN ADMINISTRATION IN SPECIAL SITUATIONS

Insulin in Hospitalized Patients

About 10% of hospitalized patients have hyperglycemia at admission. These are divided in three subgroups:
1. Known diabetics
2. Diabetes diagnosed for the first time at admission (they have raised HbA1c)
3. Stress diabetes (they have normal HbA1c)

Irrespective of the subtype they belong to, all patients with hyperglycemia at hospital admission have worse outcomes as regards, length of hospital stay, mortality, morbidity, cost of hospitalization, etc., as compared to those who are nondiabetic. Efficient management of hyperglycemia during the hospital stay helps to reduce the gap between those with hyperglycemia at admission and nondiabetics. Management of hyperglycemia during hospitalization is divided in two subgroups: (1) Management of critically ill patients and (2) management of noncritical patients admitted in wards and private rooms outside critical care.

Management of Critically Ill Patients

These patients are admitted to intensive care units and are usually not on any enteral feeding or have very unpredictable intake and poor intake through oral route or feeding tube. They often have vomiting and have wide fluctuations in their blood glucose level. Thus, they need one hourly blood glucose monitoring and a very flexible and rapid-acting antidiabetic regime. Oral antidiabetic medications have absolutely no role in critically ill patients. Even rapid-acting insulin administered through SC route is too slow to start action when the blood sugar is rising rapidly, and too slow to exit circulation when blood glucose is rapidly falling. Intravenous (IV) infusion of insulin is preferred method and is combined with 1-hourly bedside estimation of blood glucose. When insulin is administered through the IV route, the advantage of rapid-acting insulin over short-acting insulin when administered through SC route is nullified. Thus, most common type of insulin used in critically ill patients is short-acting human insulin, and administered through IV infusion. The glycemic target to be set is 140–180 mg% for critically ill medical patients and 110–140 for critically ill surgical patients. Attempts to reach more aggressive targets have resulted in a higher prevalence of hypoglycemia.

TABLE 6: Intravenous insulin infusion rate (on right) as per the prevailing blood glucose (on left).

Blood glucose (mg%)	Insulin infusion rate (U/h)
<70	off
70–109	0.2
110–119	0.5
120–149	1
150–179	1.5
180–209	2
210–239	2.5
240–269	3
270–299	3.5
300–329	4
330–359	4.5
>360	6

Intravenous infusion is made by adding 50 units of short-acting insulin into 50 mL of normal saline and infusing the mixture through an IV infusion pump. Subsequently, the bolus dose is calculated by dividing the latest blood glucose by 100 and rounding to the nearest 0.5 units of insulin and given it as IV bolus, followed by IV infusion at the same rate per hour, e.g., if prevailing blood glucose is 310 mg%, give 3 units as a bolus and then start infusion at 3 U/h. [Calculation: 310 divided by 100 = 3.1, thus the rounded bolus dose of insulin is 3 units and the rounded initial IV infusion rate is 3 units (3 mL/min through infusion pump)]. In case of nonavailability of an insulin infusion pump, add 50 units of short-acting insulin in 500 mL of normal saline and infuse at 30 mL/h. The disadvantages of this method are: (1) infusion of a larger amount of IV fluids, which could be problematic in those with impaired cardiac function and (2) inaccurate infusion rate.

After starting the infusion, do bedside blood glucose at an hourly interval and adjust the infusion rate as per **Table 6**.

If insulin infusion rate is steady for two consecutive hours, blood glucose estimation frequency is reduced to every 2 hours. If blood glucose falls below 70 mg, insulin infusion is suspended and 50 mL of 25% dextrose as bolus is infused and blood glucose estimation is repeated after 30 minutes, if blood glucose has risen to >110 mg%, insulin infusion at 50% of the last dose is started.

Conversion to Subcutaneous Insulin

Once the oral feeds are started and blood glucose is steady, shift to SC insulin. Calculate SC insulin dosage by following formula; calculate insulin infused in last 24 hours, calculate 80% of that to get TDD. About 50% of the TDD is to be injected as a daily basal insulin dose and inject it at the time of conversion. The remaining 50% is to be divided in three equal doses and injected before subsequent meals. Intravenous insulin infusion should be continued for 90 and 60 minutes respectively in those who are being converted to human insulin or analog insulin.

Note: There are multiple IV infusion protocols for critically ill patients. It is not possible to give further details in book of this size, which is primarily written for primary and secondary care clinicians. Reader is advised to refer to relevant literature.

Management of Hospitalized Noncritically Ill Patients

Noncritically ill hospitalized patients obviously have more complications, comorbidities, poorer glycemic control than ambulatory patients with diabetes, and also have more urgent need for tight glycemic control. Thus, even in those with no contraindications for the use of OADs, it is prudent to use SC insulin, unless the patients are well controlled. The type of insulin treatment plan will depend upon individual case and the basic principles are the same as those for use of insulin in ambulatory population with diabetes.

Management of Diabetes on Sick Days

Many patients omit insulin on sick days due to the misconception that their food intake is reduced considerably and, since they are vomiting, they do not require insulin and if they take it, they will develop severe hypoglycemia. However, on sick days, some patients actually require more insulin due to a rise in insulin resistance related to the underlying disease. Furthermore, vomiting and associated symptoms could be due to diabetic ketoacidosis, which is associated with severe insulin deficiency. Thus, such an arbitrary action of omitting insulin could land the patient in deep trouble. Thus, on sick days, patients should carry out frequent self-monitoring of blood glucose and urine or blood ketones and take action depending upon individual blood glucose pattern with the help of their treating doctor. They should try to prevent dehydration by taking small amounts of liquids and easily digestible soft semi solid food repeatedly under the cover of antivomiting medications. Failure of re hydration (persistent vomiting, reduced urine output, dry tongue, worsening of symptoms, etc.) is an indication for hospitalization for administration of IV fluids.

Glycemic Management during Pregnancy

Insulin is recommended as the preferred anti diabetic agent by all the guidelines for management of hyperglycemia in women with preexisting diabetes as well as gestational diabetes (GDM). Human insulin (short-acting and intermediate-acting), aspart, lispro, and detemir belong to category B (safety proved in animal studies but human studies are inadequate, though not showing any adverse effect till date) All other insulin preparations belong to category C (safety proved in animal studies but some concerns in human studies). Recently degludec was found to be noninferior to human insulin as regards safety and glycemic efficacy in a randomized study in pregnant women with diabetes and hence it may receive category B status in near future. Metformin is recommended as an alternative to insulin and also has category B status. Till 2011, glibenclamide was used as an alternative to insulin due to the then belief that it does not cross the placental barrier in significant amount. Subsequent studies with the availability of newer technology proved that placental crossing of glibenclamide was not insignificant. Furthermore, a large comparative study with insulin showed significantly higher adverse fetal outcomes with glibenclamide as compared to insulin. Thus, its use in pregnancy has declined significantly.

Points to be remembered while treating diabetes in pregnancy:
- *Glycemic goals are stringent*: FBS < 95 mg%, 1-hour postprandial glucose < 140 mg%, 2-hour postprandial glucose < 120 mg. HbA1c around 6%.
- More frequent self-monitoring is required.
- Deranged postprandial blood glucose is more strongly associated with fetal and maternal complications as compared to fasting blood glucose.
- Insulin requirement is reduced during the first trimester and gradually increases in the second and third trimester due to gradually increasing physiological insulin resistance associated with increasing levels of estrogen and progesterone.
- General principles of glycemic management with insulin in pregnancy are same as those in nonpregnant women with diabetes.

Management of Diabetes during Perioperative Period

Patients undergoing major surgery should be admitted 48–72 hours before surgery for final assessment and fine-tuning of antidiabetic therapy. In all patients who were on insulin, it should be continued.

In those type 2 diabetics with inadequate control (FBS > 150 mg%), insulin should be started. Sometimes it is advisable to start insulin in preoperative period, even in well-controlled type 2 diabetics, as insulin treatment is very flexible. These patients can be shifted back to their earlier oral antidiabetics after recovery from surgery and resuming regular oral food intake.

Three dosages of premeal short-acting/rapid-acting insulin with supplementation of long-acting or intermediate-acting insulin at bedtime for basal insulin requirement provide good round-the clock metabolic control.

If patients are on metformin, it should be discontinued 2 days prior to surgery to avoid metformin-induced lactic acidosis in perioperative period. Intraoperative or postoperative hypotension and resultant tissue hypoxia increase the chances of metformin-induced lactic acidosis. Sodium-glucose cotransporter-2 inhibitor should be discontinued 2–3 days prior to surgery to avoid euglycemic ketoacidosis. Long-acting SUs such as glibenclamide should be discontinued 2–3 days prior and short-acting SUs such as gliclazide and other agents such as repaglinide and nateglinide should be discontinued on a day prior to surgery to avoid hypoglycemia. These patients should be closely monitored for their glycemic control and appropriate insulin regime should be started to maintain glycemic control. After recovery from surgery and resumption of oral feeds and reassessing current glycemic status, OADs are reintroduced as per the prevailing glycemic situation.

ON THE DAY OF SURGERY

Fasting for at least 12 hours is required to guard against undiagnosed diabetic gastroparesis. Surgery should be scheduled in the morning session. Frequent blood glucose monitoring with reliable glucometer should be done (initially on hourly interval and subsequently on 2-hourly interval).

Glucose or glucose-insulin drip should be started in the ward before shifting the patient to the theater. 5% or 10% dextrose should be infused at the rate of 100 mL/h. In elderly or in those with left ventricular dysfunction, infusion rate should be reduced to 60–75 mL/h. Use of central line would be ideal in such situations. Daily serum electrolytes should be monitored and potassium replacement should be given accordingly till patient is stabilized and resumes his normal diet.

Insulin infusion should be given through separate microdrip, which can be "piggybacked" on dextrose drip. 55 units of short-acting human insulin should be added to a pint of normal saline. At this concentration, 10 microdrops/minute will deliver 1 U/h. The rate of microdrop infusion is to be adjusted as per the insulin requirement. If infusion pump is available, 50 units of short-acting human insulin should be added to 50 mL of normal saline and rate of infusion adjusted as per requirement (1 mL/h will deliver 1 unit of insulin/hour). Infusion pumps deliver accurate quantity of fluid and also reduce fluid overload. This is important particularly in those who require large doses of insulin and in those who have left ventricular dysfunction. Insulin requirement will depend on several factors, including degree of insulin resistance, type of surgery, state of β-cell function, etc. Insulin requirement is higher during surgeries such as CABG and renal transplantation.

Table 7 gives details about insulin infusion rates.

TABLE 7: Insulin infusion rates.	
Plasma glucose (mg%)	*Insulin infusion (U/h) or glucose bolus amount*
<70	20 mL 25% glucose bolus
71–100	1.0
101–150	1.5
151–200	2.0
201–250	3.0
251–300	4.0
>300	6.0

TABLE 8: Guidelines for selection of infusion fluid.

Blood glucose in mg%	Infusion to be administered
<100	Plain 10% glucose + KCL
101–150	10% glucose + KCL + 10 units of insulin
151–250	10% glucose + KCL + 15 units of insulin
251–300	10% glucose + KCL + 20 units of insulin
>300	Change to variable insulin infusion regimen

ALTERNATIVE INSULIN REGIMENS

- *Standard cocktail (glucose-insulin-potassium infusion)*: In standard cocktail, 10% glucose plus 15 units of short-acting insulin plus 20 mEq of potassium chloride is infused at 100 mL/h till patient resumes oral feeds. This regimen is less flexible as compared to variable rate insulin infusion described above; however, it is easier to administer. The flexibility can be increased by making four infusion sets, containing 0, 10, 15, and 20 units of insulin while keeping glucose and potassium chloride concentration fixed. Each infusion container should be labeled depending upon units of insulin mixed in it. The infusion should be selected as per blood glucose value, which should be monitored hourly during intraoperative stage and initial postoperative period, and subsequently at 2-hourly intervals. **Table 8** gives guidelines for selection of infusion fluid.
- *SC insulin*: Even though not an ideal regimen, it may be employed if IV insulin infusion regimens cannot be employed due to lack of experienced paramedical staff and resident doctors on the wards. The patient's daily insulin requirement during preoperative period is calculated. One-third of total insulin dose is given as short-acting preoperative dose subcutaneously and 5% glucose infusion is started at the rate of 100 mL/h. Blood glucose is monitored hourly and small doses (4–6 units) of short-acting insulin are given subcutaneously every 3–4 hourly if blood glucose is above 200 mg%.

MINOR SURGICAL PROCEDURES

In insulin-treated patients, SC short-acting insulin in the dose of one-third of TDD of insulin is given preoperatively and 5% glucose infusion is started at 100 mL/h. Glucose infusion is discontinued when the patient starts oral feeds and the original SC insulin regimen is reintroduced prior to first postoperative oral feed.

In patients on oral antidiabetic agents, morning pills should not be given and 5% glucose infusion should be started preoperatively and infused at 100 mL/h. Infusion should be discontinued when patient resumes oral feeds and regular oral antidiabetic drug therapy should be reintroduced simultaneously. Even in patients undergoing minor surgical procedures, fasting and preoperative, postoperative, and prefirst postoperative feed blood glucose should be estimated and the aforementioned plan should be modified if required. In stable diabetics undergoing very short procedures who are likely to resume oral feeds soon after the procedures, preoperative insulin, and immediate postoperative glucose infusion may not be required (e.g., cataract extraction, minor incision, and drainage procedures, and other procedures carried out under local anesthesia).

POSTOPERATIVE CARE

Careful monitoring of blood glucose and appropriate adjustments in insulin infusions, monitoring of vital functions, intake and urine output, and ensuring adequate hydration and at the same time avoiding over-hydration, particularly in elderly and in those with impaired left ventricular function, are important during postoperative period. Appropriate antibiotic therapy for infective conditions and prophylactic antibiotic for prevention of secondary infection in noninfective conditions are recommended. Careful and detailed attention to above mentioned points would go a long way in prevention of postoperative complications. The common postoperative complications are listed below:
- Metabolic (diabetic ketoacidosis, hyperosmolar nonketotic state, hypoglycemia, and electrolyte disturbances)
- Cardiovascular (myocardial infarction, left ventricular failure, cardiac arrhythmias, hypotension, and stroke particularly after CABG)
- Renal (acute renal failure, fluid overload)
- Infections

SPECIAL PERIOPERATIVE SITUATIONS

- *Emergency surgeries on poorly controlled patients*: Ask for 4–6 hours for critical assessment, preoperative investigations and correction of dehydration and metabolic derangement. Start the patient on IV insulin infusion and normal saline infusion through separate lines to correct hyperglycemia and fluid deficit; add potassium chloride to the pint of normal saline if there is hypokalemia. Sometimes diabetic keto acidosis presents with symptoms mimicking acute surgical abdomen. Prompt correction of hyperglycemia and fluid and electrolyte imbalance leads to rapid disappearance of symptoms. Keep this in mind when you come across the above mentioned clinical situation, insist for adequate time for correction of metabolic derangement and reassessment.
- *Coronary artery bypass graft*: Insulin requirement during intraoperative period is usually very high, 10 U/h is not uncommon. Hypothermia, liberal use of inotropic drugs and dextrose solution are some of the underlying conditions leading to high-insulin requirement.

CHAPTER 7: Insulin in the Management of Diabetes

- *Renal transplantation*: Insulin requirement is high due to infusion of large volume of fluids including dextrose, dexamethasone, and β-agonist agents. Similarly, during cesarean section the requirements of insulin go up due to β-adrenergic agonists and use of dexamethasone.

■ LONG DISTANCE AIR TRAVEL

Before embarking on long distance air travel, patients should be evaluated well in advance and the necessary insulin dose adjustments should be made and good glycemic control should be established before they begin their journey. If traveling to places in a different time zone, brief the patients and advise them as per the following guidelines.

Flying East (Days are Shorter)

- *Adjustment of basal or long-acting insulin*: (Lantus, Tresiba, Toujeo, etc.), when difference between time at departure and arrival cities is 3 hours or more.

The day before departure, give the usual dose at the usual time of day, e.g., if you are injecting 10 units of Lantus at 10 PM, take same dose at the same time on the day prior to travel.

When you begin travel, keep your watch set to your departure country time (do not change time on your watch at the start of the journey) and give half of the normal dose at the usual time, i.e., 5 units at 10 PM while in travel.

After giving this half dose, change your watch to the destination time (you can find this out from the flight attendant or from the world clock on your smartphone, googling, airline ticket (difference between time of departure and the time of arrival minus actual flying time, this information is always on your ticket, though boarding pass does not mention actual flying time. If you are wearing a smart watch such as Apple watch, it will automatically get adjusted to the arrival city time immediately after arrival).

According to your destination time, give the remaining half of the long-acting (basal) insulin at the same hour you are accustomed to giving insulin (in your case, 5 units of Lantus at 10 PM, take your Lantus at 10 PM local time at the city of arrival)

The next day keep to the destination time and give the usual full dosage at the usual time, in your case 10 units of Lantus at 10 PM local time. Give short or rapid-acting insulin before meals as usual.

Flying West (Days are Longer)

Adjustment of basal or long-acting insulin: (Lantus, Tresiba, Toujeo, etc.), when difference between time at departure and arrival cities is 3 hours or more.

The day before departure, give the usual dose at the usual time of day, in your case, 10 units of Lantus at 10 PM.

When you begin travel, keep your watch set to time of departure city and give 80–90% of regular dose at the usual time, 8 or 9 units of Lantus at 10 PM in your case. About 10% reduction if time difference is relatively short (3–4 hours, and/or current glycemic control is not very tight).

After giving this reduced dose, change your watch to the destination city time.

According to your destination time, give the usual full dose of insulin at the hour you are accustomed to (in your case 10 units of Lantus at 10 PM).

Give short- or rapid-acting insulin before meals as usual. These insulins do not require any adjustment for time zone changes, but they will require usual adjustments for food timing and amount. Since the days are longer, you will consume at more times during your flight and this will need an additional cover by injecting short or rapid-acting insulin, preferably later.

Using twice-daily premixed insulin (Mixtard, Novomix, Ryzodeg, etc.):
If you use twice-daily premixed insulin then take your usual insulin before departure at the normal time., If you are taking 10 units of Novomix before breakfast and dinner, take the last predeparture dose as usual, e.g., 10 units of Novomix before breakfast. On the flight carry a pen of rapid-acting insulin, e.g., Novorapid, Apidra, etc.). This type of insulin lasts in circulation for 3–4 hours. Check your blood glucose every 4 hours on flight. If it rises above 250 mg%, give yourself 4 units rapid-acting insulin every 4 hours (preferably with a meal), e. g., 4 units of Novorapid, until it is time for your usual second injection of premixed insulin as per destination city time after arrival, in your case 10 units of Novomix before breakfast/dinner as per the time of arrival and subsequently continue 10 units of Novomix twice-a-day before breakfast and dinner.

Please note these are simplified guideline and will need some modifications in an individual case. The key is to check your blood glucose levels frequently.

RENAL IMPAIRMENT

While endogenous insulin is metabolized by the liver, exogenous insulin is metabolized mainly by the kidneys. Thus, with advancing renal failure, insulin requirement is gradually reduced. Poor food intake due to loss of appetite, vomiting, delayed gastric emptying due to gastroparesis, reduced glycogen storage in the kidneys are some causes in addition to delayed insulin clearance, which tend to increase prevalence of hypoglycemia, while increased insulin resistance associated with renal impairment tends to push up blood glucose. Thus, the glycemic status of a given patient is extremely variable and insulin requirement cannot be predicted by the estimated glomerular filtration rate (eGFR) level alone. Moreover, there is significant day to day variability. Thus, one must rely more on rapid-acting insulin shots covering each major meal, to be administered after assessing food intake and food retention. If fasting blood glucose is not controlled by this strategy, long-acting insulin should be added at bedtime, starting with conservative dosages. This strategy should be used in severe renal impairment, while the usual strategies for the management of type 2 diabetes should be used in patients with mild renal impairment. General principle is to initiate and intensify conservatively.

INSULIN ALLERGY

Hypersensitive reactions to human insulin and insulin analogs are known to occur rarely. Often they are due to allergy to noninsulin ingredients such as protamine and expedients in the vials and cartridges. Immediate hypersensitive reactions occur within in 1 hour and consist of erythema and urticaria at the site of injection. Occasionally systemic anaphylactic reactions occur. The treatment includes withdrawal of insulin and administration of antihistamines and steroids. In patients with type 2 diabetes, one can try to maintain glycemic control with OAD combinations and GLP-1 analogs. Change of insulin formulation will be effective in those with an allergy to additives in insulin products. If these strategies do not work, insulin desensitization should be tried. Delayed hypersensitive reactions usually manifest between 6 and 24 hours in the form of local induration or nodules and generalized eczematous lesions. They tend to resolve spontaneously.

SUMMARY

Since its introduction exactly a century ago, insulin has remained on the center stage of diabetes management. Prior to the availability of exogenous insulin, diagnosis of type 1 diabetes was essentially a death certificate. While insulin products and delivery systems have dramatically improved over a period of 100 years, insulin still remains a medical necessity in all type 1 diabetic patients and is also required in many type 2 diabetic patients to reach the glycemic targets. Improvement in insulin quality and delivery systems is an ongoing process and thus, every clinician who treats diabetic patients needs to acquire working knowledge on use of insulin and constantly update it.

CHAPTER 8

Hypoglycemia with Insulin Therapy

■ INTRODUCTION

Occurrence of hypoglycemia while on insulin therapy and also fear of hypoglycemia are the main barriers in the management of diabetes. Hypoglycemia is the most common condition leading to visits to emergency rooms across the globe among all the emergencies in endocrinology practice. In the calendar year 2022, 100,000 emergency room visits were recorded in USA for the management of hypoglycemia with the mortality of 0.9 per 1,000 emergency room visits. But for hypoglycemia, therapy for diabetes would have been as simple as that of Addison's disease or hypothyroidism.

Among the antidiabetic agents, highest incidence of hypoglycemia occurs with insulin therapy and next in order are sulfonylureas and glinides; which together are called insulin secretagogues. About 90% of the patients on insulin experience at least one episode of hypoglycemia in their lifetime. The incidence of iatrogenic hypoglycemia has increased after the publication of DCCT (Diabetes Control and Complications Trial), which comprehensively proved that aggressive insulin therapy leads to tighter glycemic control which in turn reduces vascular complications of diabetes in significant manner. However, the flip side is three times higher prevalence of hypoglycemia in aggressively treated type 1 diabetes mellitus (T1DM) patients as compared to those receiving conventional treatment in DCCT.

Whenever there is a mismatch between the dosage, pharmacokinetic properties, or timing of these agents with amount, timing, and the type of food consumed and physical activity performed, hypoglycemia occurs.

Severe hypoglycemia is defined as a condition in which assistance of another person is required. Hypoglycemic coma, convulsions, and drowsiness, need to administer glucose by intravenous (IV) route, need for hospitalization, are some of the examples of severe hypoglycemia. For the diagnosis of hypoglycemia, the random blood glucose during the symptomatic stage should be 70 mg or below. Hypoglycemia can occasionally be fatal, thus should never be taken lightly.

The symptoms of hypoglycemia depend upon the rate of fall of blood glucose and the severity of hypoglycemia. The blood glucose levels at which symptoms appear are variable and depend upon previous metabolic control. In poorly controlled patients, symptoms appear at higher plasma glucose levels as compared to those who are tightly controlled. The early symptoms are known as neurogenic or autonomic symptoms because they are due to secretion of extra quantities of epinephrine, norepinephrine, and acetylcholine in the circulation as a biofeedback mechanism to control hypoglycemia. These include palpitations, tremors, anxiety, and sweating. Every patient does not get all the symptoms during the hypoglycemic episode but usually the same symptoms are present, whenever he gets hypoglycemia. These symptoms serve as a warning signal and if recognized, the patient can immediately take some carbohydrate-containing food items, such as biscuits, bread, sandwich, or sugar, to correct hypoglycemia. In milder cases, the symptoms are automatically corrected due to rise in blood glucose following secretion of extra quantities of counterregulatory hormones **(Table 1)**.

Hence, at every follow-up visit, particularly in well-controlled diabetics, the attending doctor should pointedly ask about such neurogenic symptoms, particularly before meal timings and if present, hypoglycemia should be confirmed by doing random blood glucose test at appropriate times and the dosage of insulin should be reduced appropriately. If blood glucose continues to fall further, brain is deprived of glucose—its only fuel and a new set of symptoms develop. These include hunger, headache, fainting, abnormal behavior, rowdiness, altered consciousness, and ultimately coma. Some may develop hemiparesis mimicking cerebrovascular accident while others may get convulsions. These symptoms are known as neuroglycopenic symptoms because they are due to deficiency of glucose in neurons **(Table 2)**.

In many long-standing elderly diabetics and in those who are very tightly controlled over a long period, warning neurogenic symptoms are absent and they straightaway develop neuroglycopenic symptoms. This condition

Table 1: Hormonal response during hypoglycemia.		
Glycemic threshold (mg/dL)	**Response**	**Role in prevention/correction of hypoglycemia**
80–85	↓Insulin	First defense against hypoglycemia
65–70	↑Glucagon	Primary glucose counter regulatory factor
65–70	↑Epinephrine	Critical when glucagon is deficient
65–70	↑Cortisol, growth hormone	Not critical
50–55	Symptoms	Prompt behavioral defense (food ingestion)
<50	↓Cognition	Compromises behavioral defense

Table 2: Symptoms of hypoglycemia.	
Neurogenic[1,2]	**Neuroglycopenic[1,2]**

• *Adrenergic*:
  ○ Palpitations
  ○ Tremor anxiety/arousal
• *Cholinergic*:
  ○ Sweating
  ○ Hunger paresthesia
	• Cognitive impairments
	• Behavioral changes
	• Psychomotor abnormalities
	• Seizure
	• Coma

Factors affecting glycemic thresholds are poorly controlled type 1 and type 2 diabetes mellitus, tight glycemic control in type 1 diabetes mellitus, and older age[2,3]	
Sources: 1. Cryer PE. Hypoglycemia, functional brain failure, and brain death. J Clin Invest. 2007;117(4):868-70. 2. Cryer PE, Davis SN, Shamoon H. Hypoglycemia in diabetes. Diabetes Care. 2003;26(6):1902-12. 3. Meneilly GS, Cheung E, Tuokko H. Altered responses to hypoglycemia of healthy elderly people. J Clin Endocrinol Metab. 1994;78(6):1341-8.	

is known as *"hypoglycemia unawareness"* or *"hypoglycemia-associated autonomic failure"*. Hence, every acute neuropsychiatric episode in a diabetic, on antidiabetic therapy with insulin and/or insulin secretagogue therapy (sulfonylureas and glinides such as repaglinide and nateglinide), should be treated as hypoglycemia unless proved otherwise. Those with hypoglycemia unawareness should be given higher glycemic targets to reduce frequency and severity of hypoglycemic episodes.

Whenever hypoglycemia is suspected, random blood glucose should be estimated with properly stored, valid dry strips, and periodically calibrated reliable glucometer. For confirmation of hypoglycemia in a symptomatic patient, blood glucose of 70 mg% or below should be documented and symptoms should disappear after correction of hypoglycemia. Such documentation is important, particularly in situations where symptoms are mild, recurrent, nonspecific, and if symptoms develop at times when hypoglycemia is unlikely (e.g., after meals). It is not uncommon to come across patients having many anxiety-related symptoms, which they attribute to hypoglycemia and reduce the dosage of their antidiabetic medications or even stop these medications without consulting their doctor, thus resulting in poor metabolic control.

■ REBOUND HYPERGLYCEMIA (SOMOGYI EFFECT)

It refers to hyperglycemia that follows severe hypoglycemia and can last for 12-24 hours. It is due to exaggerated and prolonged compensatory response triggered by counterregulatory hormones ("overshoot effect"). The hypoglycemic symptoms may be ignored or mild and unrecognized. Rebound hyperglycemia is often seen in patients on insulin in whom insulin dosages are increased very rapidly in an eagerness to swiftly achieve good metabolic control and in those patients in whom large dosage of insulin is given once a day, and in those patients in whom only short-acting insulin is used and fasting blood glucose control is attempted by increasing predinner dose of short-acting insulin, instead of adding intermediate-acting or long-acting insulin. Thus, it is important to remember, particularly in patients on a large dosage of insulin, that occasionally, hyperglycemia, particularly fasting hyperglycemia is due to inappropriate use of insulin and in such circumstances injecting less insulin but more frequently and using long-acting or intermediate-acting insulin to provide for basal insulinization of tissues, particularly liver will reestablish blood glucose control.

■ HYPOGLYCEMIA AFTER EXERCISE

In a normal person, aerobic exercise increases tissue sensitivity toward insulin by 20–40% at 2 hours after starting exercise and insulin release is reduced accordingly. In patients with diabetes mellitus on insulin, externally administered insulin is outside the control of biofeedback. Thus, depending upon duration and level of exercise, a diabetic patient on insulin needs to make adjustment in insulin dosage and amount and timing of food intake to avoid exercise-induced hypoglycemia. Though, occurrence of hypoglycemia within 1–2 hours after beginning of exercise is more common, it is known to occur up to 17 hours after the start of exercise. Thus, one needs to study each patient's response pattern individually by asking him to do frequent self-blood glucose estimation to study his own response pattern and adjust insulin dose and food intake accordingly. Since insulin sensitivity is likely to remain elevated for several hours, basal as well as prandial insulin dose require reduction for 24 hours after moderately heavy exercise. Once the response pattern is studied and adjustments made, repeated blood glucose estimation over and above his own set protocol is not required. Patients should be advised to consume 10–20 g of carbohydrate-based snacks every hour during prolonged exercise.

■ MANAGEMENT OF HYPOGLYCEMIA

Prevention: All diabetics on insulin and/or oral hypoglycemic agents (sulfonylureas and glinides) should receive detailed training on prevention, recognition, and management of hypoglycemia at the beginning of pharmacological treatment of hyperglycemia and they should be given repeat training at appropriate intervals which should be individualized. A person staying with the patient and caring for him should also be trained, particularly in cases of children, elderly, and cognitively impaired patients with diabetes. Patients should be asked to carry some sweets or three teaspoons of sugar or glucose in small sized "zip-lock" plastic pouches in their pocket/purse along with their diabetes identity card. They should be trained to maintain fixed-meal timing, avoid fasting, consume extra food during extra physical activity and consume a carbohydrate-containing snack or sweets in case warning neurogenic symptoms develop. After recovery from an episode of

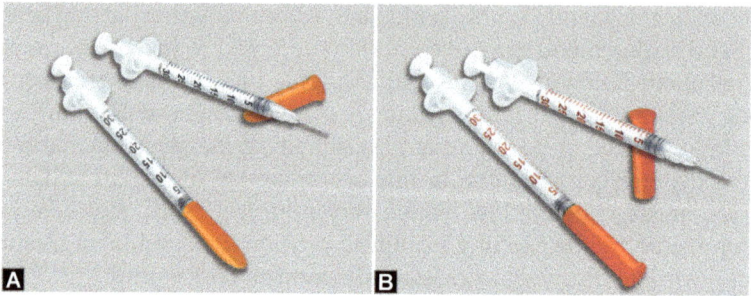

FIGS. 1A AND B: (A) U/100 syringe and (B) U/40 syringe.

hypoglycemia, the patients should critically analyze the events and identify their mistakes and correct them to avoid future hypoglycemic episodes. If hypoglycemia occurs in spite of absence of any identifiable mistake, and particularly if it is recurrent, the patients should immediately contact their doctor who will reassess the situation and appropriately reduce the dosage of their antidiabetic medications.

Patients should be trained about availability of insulin in two strengths (U/40 and U/100, containing 40 and 100 units of insulin per milliliter, respectively), and about using U/40 syringe for U/40 insulin and U/100 syringe for U/100 insulin. If U/100 insulin is filled in U/40 insulin syringe, the patient will end up receiving two and half times the intended dose and will obviously have severe hypoglycemia. This blunder is actually happening in a day-to-day practice!

Thus, patients should be encouraged to convert from syringes to pens to avoid vial-syringe mismatch. Pen use will minimize but not eliminate hypoglycemia due to mismatch because of tendency of people to "invent" cost cutting ways of insulin use. Refer to the Chapter 9 Insulin Delivery Systems, for two case reports of diabetes control going haywire due to "*jugaad*" minded patients who "manufactured" insulin cartridge by injecting insulin from U/40 vial into empty cartridge resulting in severe hyperglycemia while in other case, where a patient withdrew insulin from cartridge, filled it in U/40 syringe and injected it resulting in repeated hypoglycemia.

- U/100 insulin syringes have orange caps and black marks and figures.
- U/40 insulin syringes have red caps and red marks and figures (**Figs. 1A and B**).

■ TREATMENT OF SEVERE HYPOGLYCEMIA

If the patient is conscious and alert, he should be asked to take three teaspoons, 15 g of sugar or glucose. If there is no improvement in symptoms or if repeat blood glucose is not >100 mg% at 15 minutes, he should repeat three teaspoons of sugar and wait for another 15 minutes. If there is no recovery in another 15 minutes or worsening of symptoms or persistence of blood glucose >100 mg%, medical attention should be sought. If he is unconscious, drowsy or rowdy, 50 mL of 25% glucose should be given as IV bolus. In case a patient is on long-acting sulfonylurea, such as glibenclamide, IV bolus of 25% glucose should be followed by a pint of 5% glucose, which should be continued till his blood glucose is stabilized. These patients can have a prolonged or recurrent hypoglycemia and thus require close observation and repeated blood glucose estimations up to 48 hours. If IV access is difficult, 1 mg of glucagon should be injected subcutaneously or intramuscularly. For children weighing <20 kg, the dose is 0.5 mg. The relatives of patients prone to get severe hypoglycemia, particularly those who do not have warning hypoglycemic symptoms, should be instructed to keep a vial of glucagon handy and inject it during hypoglycemic emergency. Immediately after the injection patient should be nursed on his sides to reduce chances of aspiration in case of vomiting. "Ready for injection" glucagon and nasal glucagon spray are now available in USA but the cost is prohibitive. Please note that glucagon is not freely available in our country.

The management of diabetes is a balancing act between tight glycemic control and episodes of hypoglycemia. Tighter the control, lesser the complications: but, at the cost of higher chances of hypoglycemia as clearly shown in the graph **(Fig. 2)**. The treating clinician should be shrewd and experienced to set individual goals depending upon variables, such as age, comorbid conditions, life expectancy, patient's attitude, and support system and then achieve the goal by carefully selecting appropriate insulin formulation to suit individual needs; and giving detailed education about lifestyle from the point of view of avoiding hypoglycemia **(Fig. 3)**. As regards hypoglycemia prevalence, rapid-acting insulin analogs have advantage over short-acting insulin while long-acting analog insulin formulations have definite advantage over intermediate-acting insulin.

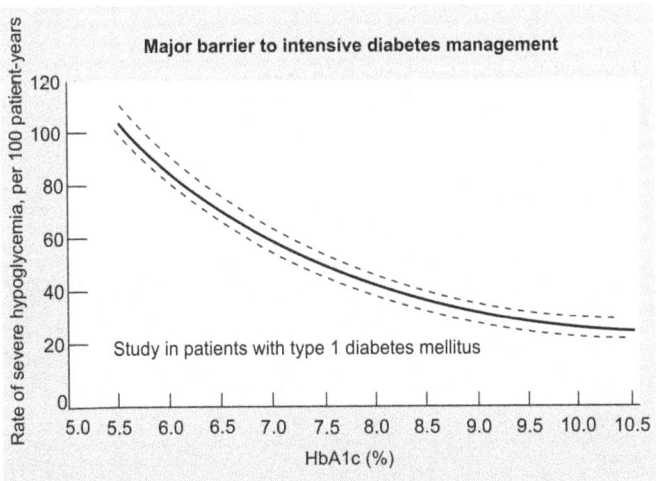

FIG. 2: Rates of severe hypoglycemia increase as glycated hemoglobin (HbA1c) levels decrease in patients with diabetes.

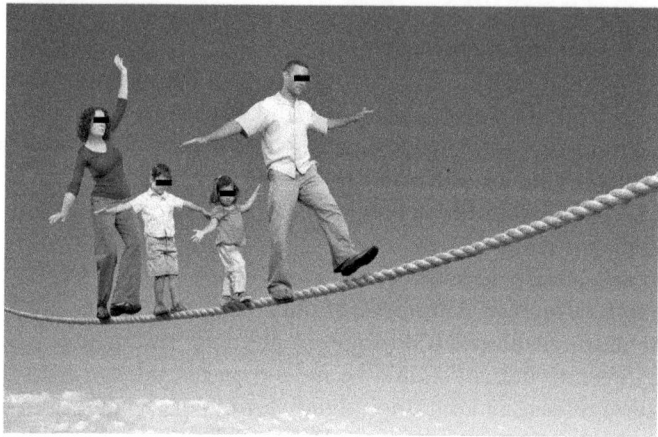

FIG. 3: The management of diabetes is balancing tight glycemic control and hypoglycemia.

SUMMARY

Hypoglycemia and fear of hypoglycemia are the major stumbling blocks in the way of achieving desired glycemic control in the management of diabetes. Thus, a clinician should acquire in-depth knowledge and experience to minimize hypoglycemic episodes in the patients they put on insulin therapy, and also develop skills to educate the patients as regards ways and means of minimizing hypoglycemic episodes and to remove fear of hypoglycemia from their minds so as to increase their compliance for insulin therapy, which is a vital necessity for achieving glycemic targets. The availability of rapid-acting and ultra rapid-acting insulin analogs as well as long-acting insulin analogs in the recent past have definitely made the task much easier.

CHAPTER 9

Insulin Delivery Systems

■ INTRODUCTION

Therapeutically, insulin is delivered through subcutaneous (SC) route for routine use and through intravenous (IV) route during emergencies and critical states. In this chapter, we will be mainly discussing the available options for SC insulin delivery. In addition, inhaled insulin for prandial use as an alternative for rapid-acting insulin is available in dry powder form in USA. It is inhaled through a small device.

Insulin is delivered SC in three different ways:
1. *Insulin vials*: Through dedicated plastic insulin syringes with fixed needles. Several brands are available in the market. The brand sold most commonly is BD syringes. They are available in two versions, U/40 as well as U/100. The needles are 6 mm long and have bore of 31G size and are fixed to the syringes. The plunger has non latex flat rubber at the end and no dead space. U/40 syringes have red cap and red markings and dosage numbers, while U/100 syringes have orange cap, black markings, and dosage numbers. While the former is meant for drawing insulin from U/40 vials, the latter is to be used to draw insulin from U/100 vials. The needles are presterilized and disposable, meant for single use. When prescribing insulin formulation in vial form, please train the patients and their caregivers in details and verify the purchases made by them to ensure that there is no vial-syringe mismatch.
2. *Insulin pens*: The first insulin pen for SC insulin administration was introduced in 1985. Since then, there has been a continuous improvement in the quality and user-friendly nature of insulin pens. The pens in current use have patient-friendly features, such as easily readable dosage window, audible click at the end of complete dosing, requirement of minimal force for pushing the plunger, and facility for dose resetting. Today, a large majority of patients prefer insulin pens over insulin syringes. The pens are available in two formats, (1) disposable pens and (2) reusable pens. Disposable pens are preloaded with insulin cartridge inside a sealed

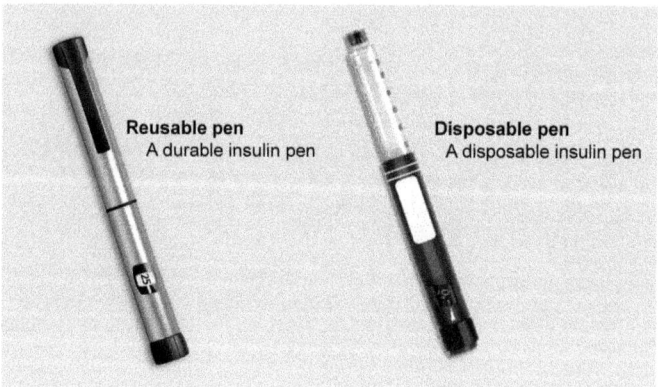

FIG. 1: Reusable insulin pen on the left and disposable pen on the right.

compartment. They are in "ready to use" form, but once all the insulin (300 units) is used up, these pens cannot be refilled. In reusable pens, one needs to replace the insulin cartridge, just like one replaces the ball pen refills **(Fig. 1)**. When one is expected to use insulin for a short-term or if one wants to try out the suitability of pens, he should be advised to use disposable pens. Long-term insulin users are advised to use reusable pens, as it is less expensive to use them as compared to disposable pens. The maximum one-time cost of reusable pen is approximately ₹1,500/. The insulin analogs are usually available only in pen forms, with the exception of Lantus, (glargine 100) and Novorapid, which are also available in conventional vial form (U/100 only). With little bargaining, reusable insulin pens can be obtained free of cost (insulin in cartridge form has better margin, thus companies can afford to give free reusable pens if the user is expected to use them, and thus their insulin cartridges for a long term). Detachable and single-use 32 bore 4-mm long needles are to be attached to these pens before the delivery of insulin.

3. *Insulin pumps*: Several models of portable insulin pumps, which can be strapped onto the abdominal wall, are in day-to-day use. A needle that is inserted in the SC tissue on the anterior abdominal wall and secured with an adhesive tape is connected to the other end of the pump via polyethylene tubing. The pump case contains a syringe, the piston of which is driven by the pump. The rate of continuous insulin delivery is adjustable. In addition, there is a provision to give a premeal booster dose of insulin. By using the pump, it is possible to deliver insulin in continuous SC infusion at a rate mimicking the physiological rate of insulin delivered from the pancreas. For more than three decades, a large number of patients, mostly type 1 diabetes mellitus (T1DM) patients, have been using these pumps and it has been shown that their use leads to a lesser incidence of hypoglycemic episodes; and a better control of blood glucose level, thus postponing specific complications of diabetes

as compared to conventional insulin administration. However, pumps administer insulin into the systemic circulation and not into the portal circulation. This delivery system has its limitations described in details elsewhere. Another drawback of the open-loop system is the absence of an algorithm to automatically determine the insulin dosage, based on the data provided by the sensor, and coordinate with the pump to deliver it. The currently available pumps in a day-to-day practice belong to an open-loop system, i.e., the decisions about insulin dosage and dosage administration are manual. The pumps belonging to closed loop system are called artificial pancreas. In these pumps, the dosage algorithm is integrated into the system and most of the dosage changes, except the determination of prandial bolus dosages, are algorithm driven. About a year back, the first artificial pancreas received permission in the USA for introduction in day-to-day practice. The truly complete artificial pancreas is still in the experimental stage.

The complications and limitations of insulin pumps include equipment failure leading to too much or too little insulin administration with obvious consequences, cutaneous complications such as painful lumps and abscesses at the site of needle insertion, which are not very rare, and initial and recurring cost—the cost of pumps (minimum ₹100,000/- and ₹4,000/- respectively) is out of reach of average Indians. However, a number of Indian diabetic patients using pumps have gone up significantly over the last decade.

■ INDICATIONS FOR INSULIN PUMPS

Patients having T1DM and some with type 2 diabetes mellitus (T2DM) on insulin therapy, particularly those with brittle diabetes, those having frequent hypoglycemic episodes, those opting for more flexible lifestyle, and those wanting to reduce daily prick, are the candidates for insulin administration through the pumps. However, one should have pragmatic expectations of the pumps. Glycemic control will be better but short of ideal in most. Similarly, hypoglycemic episodes will be lesser, but not totally eliminated.

Recently, an upgraded version of the conventional insulin pump has been developed. It contains an inbuilt sensor to continuously monitor glucose levels. The glucose data is fed into the pump's memory and it automatically stops delivery of insulin for a specified period of time if the interstitial fluid glucose level dips below 70 mg%, thus preventing hypoglycemia. This is a big step forward over stand-alone sensors that are in use for more than a decade and pumps with inbuilt sensors in a system that are not smart to suspend insulin delivery during impending hypoglycemia.

When to use Insulin Vials and When to use Insulin Pens?

The traditional method of injecting insulin consists of using disposable plastic insulin syringes, which are used to draw insulin from the glass vials as well as to inject insulin into the patient's body. This is the least expensive way of injecting insulin but a bit more time-consuming, cumbersome, a bit more painful and less accurate method as compared to injecting insulin through insulin pens. Injecting insulin through pens is less time-consuming and more convenient. In addition, the dosing is precise. The upper portion of pen is rotated in a clockwise manner till the numerical figure of insulin dose appears in a window at its upper end. This is known as "dialing of dose". In short, insulin pens are a smarter and more convenient option. Besides the abovementioned comparative advantages of pens over syringes, the former provide more privacy and thus are more acceptable and have better patient adherence and thus provide better glycemic control. In addition, the patient is protected from severe glycemic derangement due to mismatch between vials and syringes. Thus, pens are cost-effective over a long-term period due to reduction in hospitalization rates.

The patients opting for economy should be advised to continue injecting insulin with syringes. Patients requiring >40 units of insulin at a time should be prescribed U/100 insulin vials and syringes in order to avoid extra pricks (the capacity of U/40 syringe is 40 units). The additional advantage of using insulin from U/100 vial is reduced volume of injected insulin, which is less painful.

How to Avoid Mistakes while Injecting/Prescribing Insulin?

Mistakes due to mismatch between insulin vials and syringes—some real-life "comic mistakes" leading to tragic implications:

Today, the most common mode of administration of insulin is through SC route by using insulin syringes. Looking at rapid economic development of our country, very aggressive strategies of insulin marketing companies to encourage shift from syringes to pens (margins are higher in cartridges and regulated by the government for vials) and rapid conversion rate in the last few years, this situation will change sooner than later but clinicians have to be alert. After having prescribed insulin injections, it is the prescribing doctor's duty to ensure that the prescription bears all the details such as units and type of insulin, its frequency, the time gap between injection and food intake, vial strength, and specifications of insulin syringe. Insulin vials are available in two strengths: (1) U/40 and (2) U/100, containing 40 units and 100 units, respectively, per each milliliter. Insulin syringes are also available in two types: (1) U/40 and (2) U/100, each made specifically to suit specific insulin vial. Besides teaching proper insulin injection techniques, it is advisable that the treating doctor also briefs them about different vial strengths and syringe types. He should advise them to always verify the vial strength whenever a new vial is to be used and to draw insulin in matching syringes. However, in a day-to-day practice, occasionally, major mistakes occur, either due to lack of time available at the doctor's disposal or because of carelessness of the patient. These mistakes in insulin injection technique lead to hypoglycemia or hyperglycemia as per individual mistake. Sometimes, life-threatening emergencies are created. Some of the actual mistakes the author has come across have been described below:

- A patient was taking injection Huminsulin (30/70) (U/40 vial) 40 units twice a day and his blood glucose was poorly controlled, thus he was advised to use injection Huminsulin (30/70) 50 units twice a day. Since the capacity of U/40 syringe is only 40 units, he was advised to use a U/100 syringe so that "you can take up to 50 unit mark and avoid two pricks". The patient followed the advice and his blood glucose further worsened. At this point, he consulted us. The reason for worsening of blood glucose was obvious. If one takes U/40 insulin up to the 50 unit mark in a U/100 syringe, he actually takes only 20 units. So, instead of increasing insulin from 40 to 50 units, he ended up reducing it to 20 units.

> *Take home message*: In such situations, instruct the patient to change over to a U/100 vial as well as U/100 insulin syringe, or to change over to insulin pens.

- An uneducated patient taking injection of Mixtard (30/70) 48 units, before breakfast and 34 units before dinner came to the outpatient department alone. His blood glucose levels were high. His compliance with insulin injections was apparently good, so was his diet control. He was investigated for lack of blood glucose control in spite of an apparent high dose of insulin. He could not answer questions regarding the type of insulin syringe. However, when asked about the cost of insulin vial, he could answer the question correctly and from this information, we derived that he was taking U/40 insulin. When asked, "how long will the bottle last"? We found that his bottle was lasting 2.5 times the expected period. From this data, we concluded that he was taking U/40 insulin with a U/100 syringe, thus actually taking only 40% of the prescribed dose. We asked him to come back with a vial and syringe and confirmed the same. When he changed over to U/40 syringe, his blood glucose was controlled.

> *Take home message:* If your patient's blood glucose is not well controlled in spite of good compliance, always find out from him how many days the vial lasts. If vial is lasts for much longer than expected (around 2.5 times), suspect the mismatch between insulin vial and syringe (specifically, suspect that patient is injecting insulin from a U/40 vial with a U/100 syringe. For example, if your patient is prescribed 20 units of insulin twice a day, he will finish the vial in exactly 10 days. Each vial contains 400 units of insulin: 40 units/mL in a 10 mL vial). However, if he uses a U/100 syringe and draws insulin up to the 20 unit mark, he will end up using only 8 units of insulin at a time, or 16 units per day. Thus, vial will last for 25 days.

- Many of the patients have friends or relatives in the USA. Whenever these nonresident Indian relatives know that their India-based kin is on insulin injections, they send a large carton containing disposable insulin syringes. These are invariably U/100 syringes, which are designed to inject U/100 insulin, the only strength of insulin available for common use in the entire developed world. However, in India, even though both the strengths of insulin are available, 99 out of 100 times the patient is on U/40 strength. Thus, if insulin from U/40 vials is drawn up in U/100 syringes, patients end up injecting only 40% of the prescribed dose, unless they draw 2.5 times the prescribed dose in the syringe. Thus, it is better to avoid using a U/100 syringe for U/40 insulin injection. However, in an emergency, one may multiply the prescribed dose by 2.5 times and use U/100 syringe for U/40 insulin. For example, if one is prescribed 20 units of insulin and usually uses U/40 vials and U/40 syringes, if he has to use a U/100 syringe, he should withdraw insulin from a U/40 vial up to the 50 unit mark in U/100 syringe.

On the other hand, in the case of an extremely rare situation of needing to inject U/100 insulin with a U/40 syringe, one has to multiply by a factor of 0.4. For example, if one is prescribed 20 units of insulin and is usually uses U/100 vials with U/100 syringes, if he has to use a U/40 syringe, he should draw insulin from a U/100 vial up to the 8 unit mark on U/40 syringe (U/40 syringes have red top and are marked up to 40 in red, while U/100 syringes have orange top and are marked up to 100 in black). In order to find out the strength of an insulin vial, ask the questions regarding the cost of vials to get the information. U/40 vial costs between ₹125/- and ₹150/-, while a U/100 vial obviously costs more than ₹300/-.

- A patient was taking 40 units of Huminsulin (30/70) in the morning and 20 units in the evening. His fasting blood glucose (FBG) was well controlled but postlunch blood glucose was high, thus his morning dose was increased to 44 units while no change was made in evening dose. Since one can only take up to 40 units of insulin in a U/40 syringe, he was rightly advised to change over to a U/100 insulin vial and inject it with a U/100 insulin syringe. However, he continued to take an evening dose of 20 units from a U/40 vial and with a U/40 syringe and ordered fresh stocks of U/40 vial and syringes even after the vial in use was finished.

  He did not make any technical mistakes, but after using all the remaining insulin from the U/40 vial for the evening dose, he could have taken 20 units in the evening from the U/I00 vial which he was using for the morning. There was no need to keep inventory of two vials and two types of syringes.

  > *Take home message*: You can use U/100 insulin vials and syringes for small as well as large doses, but you cannot inject >40 units of U/40 insulin with a U/40 syringe.
  >
  > Thus, always match insulin vial strength with the insulin syringe.

- A 45-year-old female patient, whose blood glucose was not controlled in spite of triple drug oral combination, was put on Mixtard (30/70) 8 units each before breakfast and dinner. She was a resident of a village on the mainland about 50 km across island city of Mumbai, and was in a hurry to catch the last launch, thus she skipped the training session for insulin injections, which we hold for all patients requiring insulin for the first time. On reaching the shore, around dinner time, she approached a "trainee nurse" in a private nursing home in her village and the patient's husband literally forced the nurse to give her insulin, even though the nurse was reluctant. Under pressure, the "nurse" accepted the proposal and injected an entire vial containing 10 mL or 400 units through a 10 mL conventional multipurpose syringe. Patient walked 1.5 km to reach home and subsequently developed symptoms of hypoglycemia. Her husband immediately contacted me and narrated the incident. She was advised to be shifted to a nursing home immediately. She was kept in the nursing home for 48 hours under constant IV glucose infusion and a dire life-threatening emergency was avoided. Faulty technique leading to partial injection and poor absorption from a large SC deposit could have contributed to some extent. The availability of mobile phones saved her life. This was my first experience with emergency lifesaving teleconsultation about 20 years back.

> *Take home message*: It is prescribing doctor's duty to ensure safe administration of insulin to his patients and nothing should be taken for granted.

- A patient was prescribed 10 units of Huminsulin (30/70) (U/40) before dinner. She was well controlled with appropriate syringes and vials purchased from the market, till she received a vial of Huminsulin (30/70) (U/100) free of cost from her employer's medical services department. Nobody briefed her about the difference between U/40 and U/100 vials and the need to use appropriate syringes. For a few days, she used U/40 syringe to inject insulin from U/100 vials. One fine day, the family doctor, who used to come to visit her daily for injecting insulin, noticed that he was drawing U/100 insulin in U/40 syringe. He decided to draw up to 25 unit mark to account for the difference (he should have drawn up to 4 unit mark). Thus, he injected 62.5 units subcutaneously. In other words, he magnified the mistake 2.5 times. The patient developed severe hypoglycemia.

> *Take home message*: All patients on insulin, their relatives who are involved in their care, and their primary care medical and paramedical personnel, all should receive intensive education on the availability of insulin vials and syringes in different strengths. As far as possible, do not use inappropriate syringes to avoid calculation mistakes. Use of insulin pens, which almost completely eliminates this problem, should be encouraged.

- A 43-year-old female patient was put on injection of Mixtard (30/70) 20 units before breakfast and dinner with reusable pen, and had stable

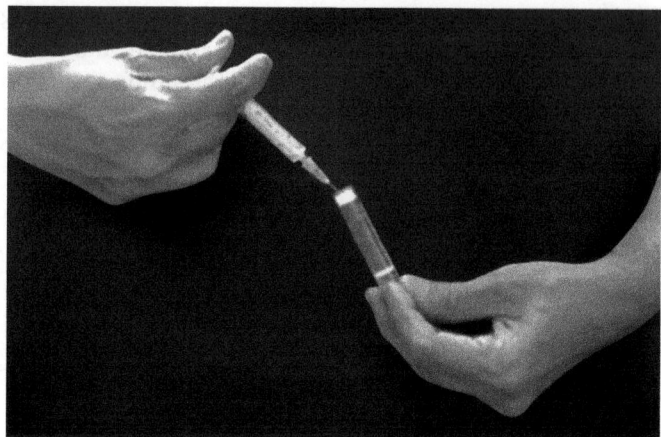

FIG. 2: Faulty improvisation: Patient filling empty Mixtard cartridge by injecting Mixtard, drawn from U/40 vial, through rear-end of cartridge.

blood glucose control till she decided to do cost cutting by purchasing Mixtard (30/70) U/40 vial from the market and by refilling empty Mixtard cartridges via syringe filled with insulin drawn from Mixtard U/40 vial. Soon her blood glucose rose significantly. The reason is obvious. While a Mixtard cartridge contains 100 units/mL, Mixtard U/40 from vial contains 40 units/mL. Thus, the patient ended up taking only 8 units of insulin twice a day instead of 20 units twice a day.

Figure 2 depicts how the patient improvised by refilling insulin cartridge from its rear end by injecting Mixtard drawn from a U/40 vial.

- A 56-year-old female was admitted under us for the management of severely infected diabetic foot. As per the history obtained at admission, she was on 12 units of Mixtard 30/70 before breakfast and dinner. We continued same dose of insulin on day 1 and monitored her whole blood capillary glucose five times daily as per our hospital protocol. We found that her blood glucose values were in low normal to mild hypoglycemia range. On detailed interrogation of her husband, who used to inject insulin in her, we found that he was initially using reusable pens for injection and they had built up a stock of few extra cartridges. In order to use them up before expiry, the husband purchased U/40 BD insulin syringes and every time at the time of injection, drew insulin from the cartridge up to 12 mark on the U/40 syringe, pulled it out and injected insulin in his wife's SC tissue. Thus, he ended up injecting 30 units every time and the cat was out of the bag. The reasons of her hypoglycemia became clear.

  Now you will understand why I wrote that the shift from vials and syringes to pens "will almost completely eliminate" the mismatch problems, instead of writing will "completely eliminate" the problem.

- A 66-year-old female patient was prescribed 15 units of Mixtard (30/70) before breakfast. She went to a small chemist shop in the by-lanes of

Mumbai for purchasing insulin vial and syringes. Chemist gave her U/100 vial and U/40 syringes. She was regularly taking "15 units of insulin" daily before breakfast and was occasionally experiencing hypoglycemic episodes. At this stage, she came to us for second opinion. We asked her to come back with her insulin vial and syringe for verification and identified her mistake.

Her mistake was explained in details and she was trained to change over to U/40 vials and draw 15 units of insulin in U/40 syringe for injection. An elaborate prescription with highlighting of relevant portion was handed over to her. Her young daughter was also briefed in details.

> *Take home message*: Do not take anything for granted. Do not rely on patients. Verify each step. In case of doubt, physically inspect the vials and syringes.

- *A mistake which luckily turned out to be beneficial*: A 43-year-old male, a known diabetic for 3 years, was hospitalized for anterior wall infarction. He was on IV insulin infusion for 48 hours and was subsequently discharged on 10 units of Mixtard before breakfast and dinner. He was prescribed U/40 insulin with U/40 insulin syringes. When he came for follow-up after 6 weeks, his fasting and postlunch plasma glucose values were 100 mg% and 132 mg%, respectively.

    Everything was apparently OK. However, on routine verification drive, it was found out that the vials of insulin were lasting much longer than expected. On further investigations, it was found out that he was using U/100 syringe for injection of U/40 strength insulin, thus effectively, he was taking only 4 units of premixed (30/70) insulin twice a day and still his blood glucose was well controlled. Subsequently, his insulin was discontinued and he was kept on aggressive lifestyle measures and when he came for follow-up after 4 weeks, his fasting and postlunch plasma glucose values were 96 mg% and 130 mg%, respectively. Thus, in his case, if he had taken insulin correctly as advised, he would have landed into hypoglycemia. His insulin requirement probably went down faster than anticipated due to disappearance of transient insulin resistance associated with acute myocardial infarction.

    > *Take home message*: Even in those patients apparently doing very well, do not take things for granted and verify compatibility between insulin vials and syringes.

- *Double mistakes also happen*: A 65-year-old woman, having T2DM for 10 years with grossly uncontrolled blood glucose in spite of three oral antidiabetic drugs (OADs), was prescribed injection Huminsulin (30/70) 10 units before breakfast and dinner. The most reputed chemist of the area having a few practicing diabetologists and several consultant physicians in his drainage area filled the prescription by supplying U/40 Mixtard vial and U/100 insulin syringe. The vial and syringe were carried to her family doctor who administered the insulin injection twice a day for 10 days with syringes carried by the patient. Thus, the patient ended up taking only 4 units of insulin twice a day, which was 40% of the prescribed dose. Thus, after 10 days, when she repeated her blood glucose levels, they were only marginally better than baseline. The mistake was identified at first follow-up. The problem was overlooked at two stages: the chemist and the family doctor.

> *Take home message*: Do not take anybody for granted. Specifically mention vial strength and syringe subtype as a suffix after insulin and syringe prescription, respectively.

Within hours after sending the final proofs to the publisher, I came across the following interesting case of severe hyperglycemia due to mismatch between insulin syringe and vial strengths. In this case, the mistake of the manufacturer of the syringes, or possibly their change in policy regarding color coding of syringe caps, or the availability of syringes manufactured by the third party getting the access to the market clandestinely was the driving cause leading to the mishap.

After experiencing several types of mismatches between vials and syringes and blunders while using the cartridges, I had a firm belief that I had seen all the possible cases. Thus, I was totally surprised to come across a case leading to severe hyperglycemia following a totally unexpected variety of mismatch.

A 66-year-old lady, having diabetes for a long time and being treated with Injection Mixtard 50/50, 32 units before breakfast and 20 units before dinner came for a regular follow-up. Her fasting and postbreakfast blood glucose values were 203 and 419 mg%, respectively. At previous follow-up, her corresponding blood glucose values were 134 and 211 mg%, respectively, while on the same dose of Mixtard 50/50. She was trained on insulin syringe–vial compatibility by verification of the following three points: (1) color of the syringe cap (red for U/40 and orange for U/100), (2) color of lettering and markings on the syringe (red for U/40 and black for U/100), and (3) units mentioned at the bottom of the syringe (40 for U/40 and 100 for U/100). The patient and her son, who closely supervised all her diabetes management-related activities, had decided to concentrate on verification by the color of syringe cap, undoubtedly the most prominent distinguishing feature between U/40 and U/100 syringes. When we suspected a vial–syringe mismatch, we closely inspected her current insulin vial and syringe, and *the cat was out of the bag* [she was drawing insulin from a U/40 vial through a U/100 syringe (black-colored numbers up to 100)]. The mistake occurred in spite of verifying the suitability of the syringe from the cap color, because it had a red cap instead of the usual orange cap **(Fig. 3)**. Thus, she was injecting only 40% of the prescribed dose. This was the cause of severe hyperglycemia.

CHAPTER 9: Insulin Delivery Systems

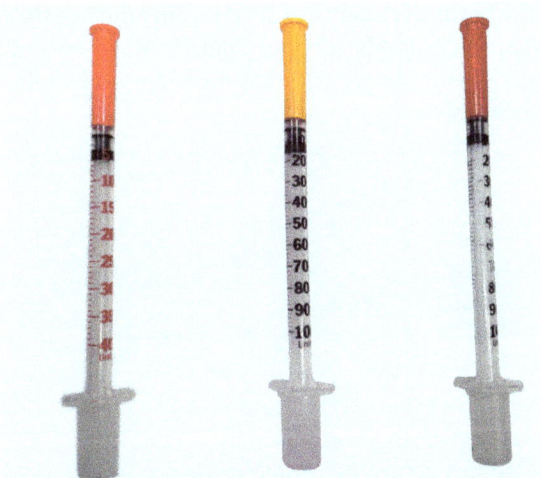

FIG. 3: U/40 and U/100 insulin syringes. Left: U/40 syringe; Center: Usual U/100 syringe with orange cap; Right: The syringe which the patient was using. Note: U/100 syringe with red cap but black lettering up 100.

> *Take home message*: As regards verifying the suitability of insulin syringes for the prescribed strength of insulin, train and retrain the patients at periodic intervals to verify all the three distinguishing features between the two types of insulin syringes.

All the cases described above are 100% real cases, none of them are imaginary. However, the very encouraging news is that of late I am getting a significantly fewer number of such cases, indicating that there is a vast improvement in insulin administration-related knowledge among patients, caregivers and medical and paramedical staff. Additionally, a larger percentage of patients shifting to insulin pens has helped.

▌ MIXING INSULIN AND INJECTING INSULIN

- Thoroughly wash your hands, cleanliness is important and helps prevent infections.

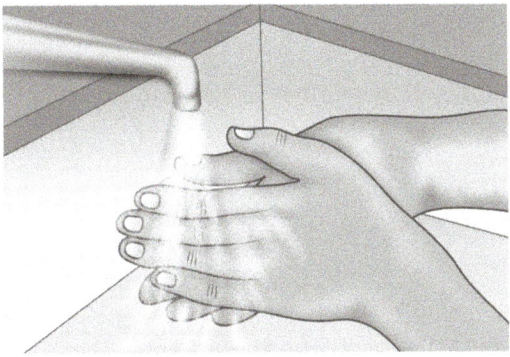

- Slowly roll the bottle of cloudy insulin (Huminsulin N, Mixtard, Insulatard, etc.) between your hands (do not shake). Make sure that the cloudy insulin is mixed completely and that there are no insulin crystals at the bottom of the bottle.

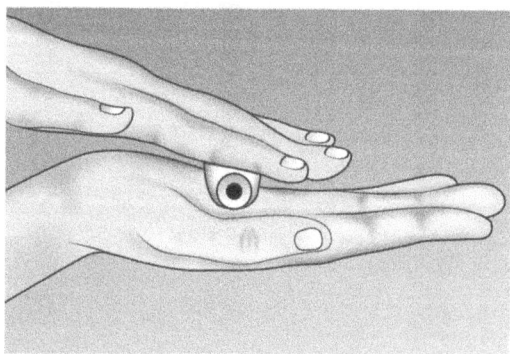

- Clean the rubber stopper of each bottle with spirit swab. For example, we are going to draw a total of 30 units of insulin, 20 units of cloudy insulin, and 10 units of regular (crystalline/plain) insulin (e.g., Huminsulin R, Actrapid).

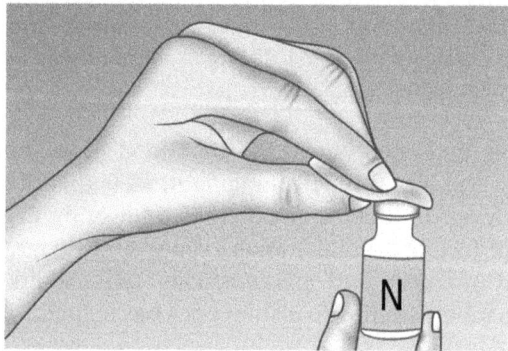

- First, draw air into the syringe to the dose of cloudy insulin. In our example, it is 20 units.

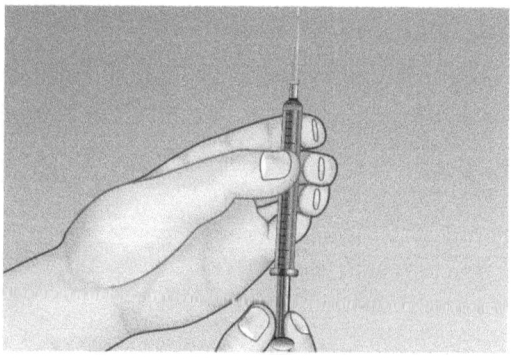

- Insert the needle through the stopper of the bottle of cloudy insulin and push 20 units of air into the bottle. Keep the bottle upright and remove the syringe. Do not draw any of the cloudy insulin yet.

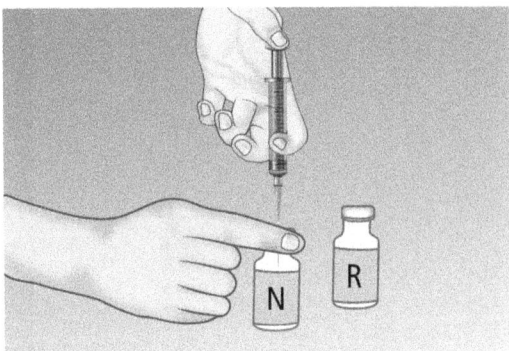

- Now fill the syringe with air equal to the number of units of clear insulin, i.e., 10 units. Insert the needle through the stopper of the regular insulin bottle and push the air into the bottle by pushing on the plunger.

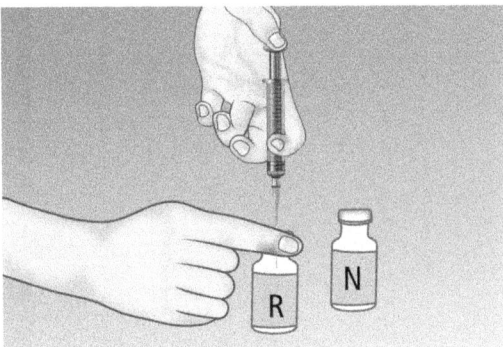

- Leave the needle in the bottle. Turn the bottle upside down. Pull down on the plunger to draw about 15 units of clear insulin, 5 more units than the 10 units we are using for our example.

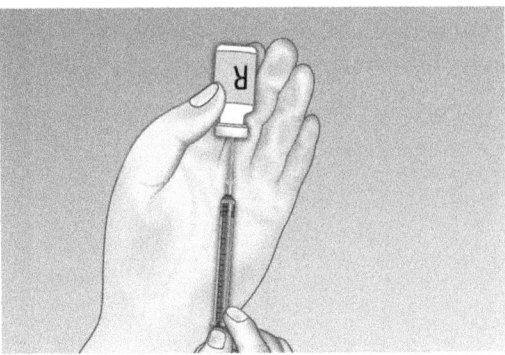

- To remove any air bubbles in the syringe, flick or tap the syringe at the site of the bubbles. This will push the bubbles to the top of the syringe. Push up on the plunger to force the bubbles back into the bottle.

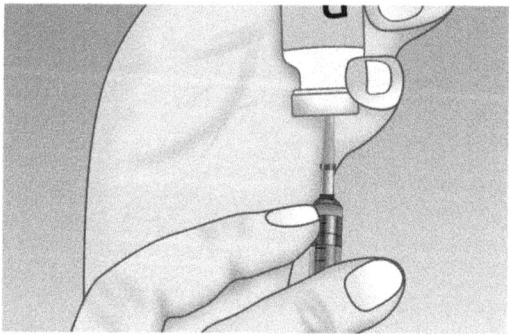

- With the needle still in the bottle, hold it up to the light and recheck it for air bubbles. If there are no air bubbles in your syringe, push the plunger to the 10 unit mark. Although, this air is not dangerous if injected, you should remove the bubbles from the syringe so that your insulin dose is accurate.

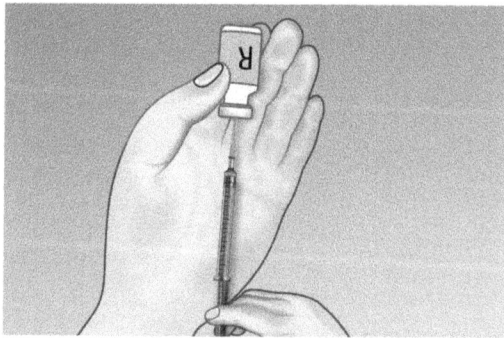

- Holding the bottle upside down, put the needle through the stopper of the cloudy insulin. For this example, we are using 20 units of cloudy insulin. Since you already have 10 units of clear insulin in the syringe, you will pull the plunger out to the mark showing 30 units, the total of the two types of insulin. Remove the needle with the syringe from the bottle.

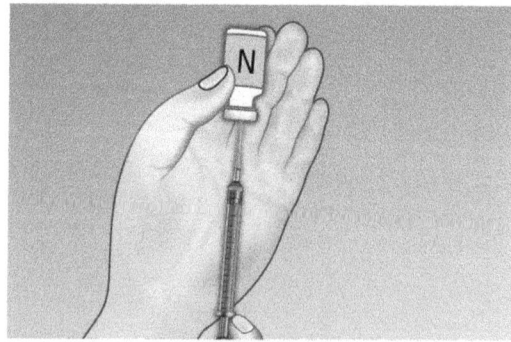

Check again for bubbles. It is rare to see them at this step, but if you do, discard this syringe and start again at step 1.

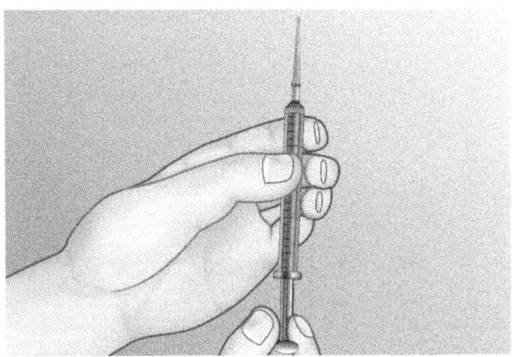

Correct Technique for Self-injection
- Wash your hands thoroughly with soap and water and apply spirit or isopropyl alcohol (which is available at the chemist) to the skin at the site of injection. Wait for a minute for the spirit/alcohol to dry up.

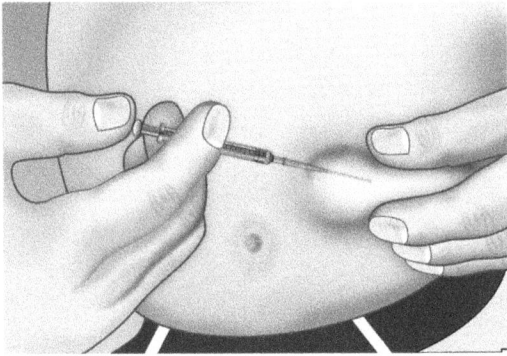

- Grip the syringe and with the other hand, pinch up a mound of skin.

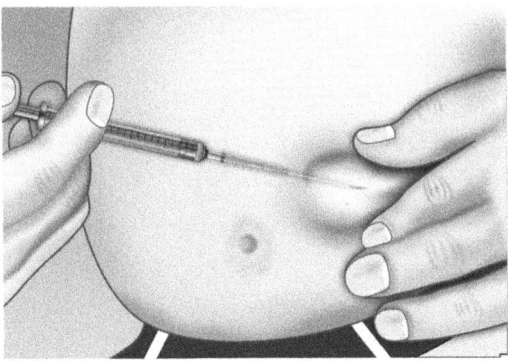

- Hold the syringe at an angle of 60° to the skin.

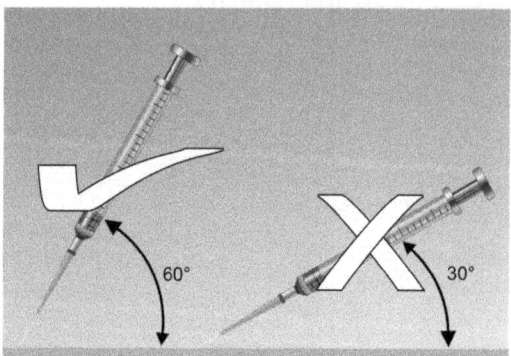

- Press the skin gently with the needle so that it "dimples".

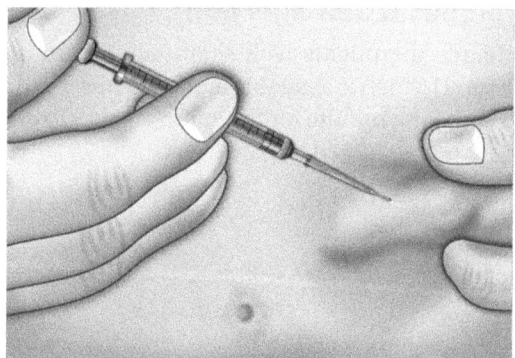

- Insert the needle to its full length.

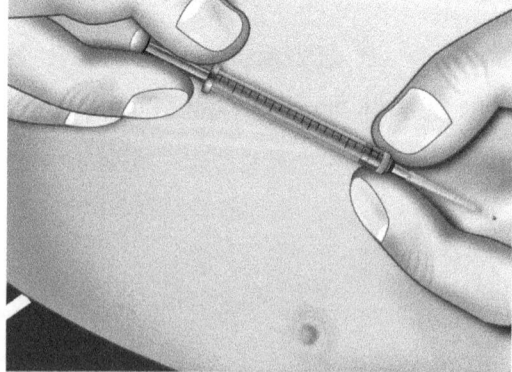

- Let go the skin and grasp the lower end of the syringe.

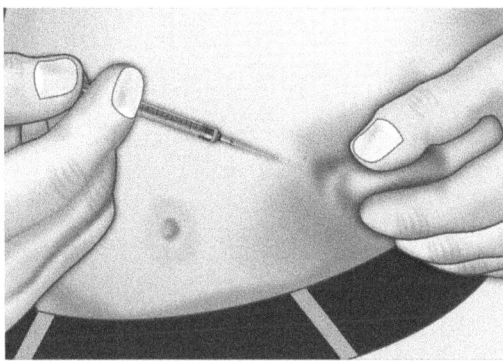

- With the other hand, gently raise the plunger a little way. If blood appears in the syringe, withdraw the needle and start again. If no blood appears, place your thumb on top of the plunger and inject insulin.
- Quickly withdraw the needle and press firmly over the injection site with a clean dry cotton swab for a few seconds. Do not rub.

Stepwise Procedure for Using Reusable Insulin Pen

1. Pull off the pen cap. Unscrew the pen apart.

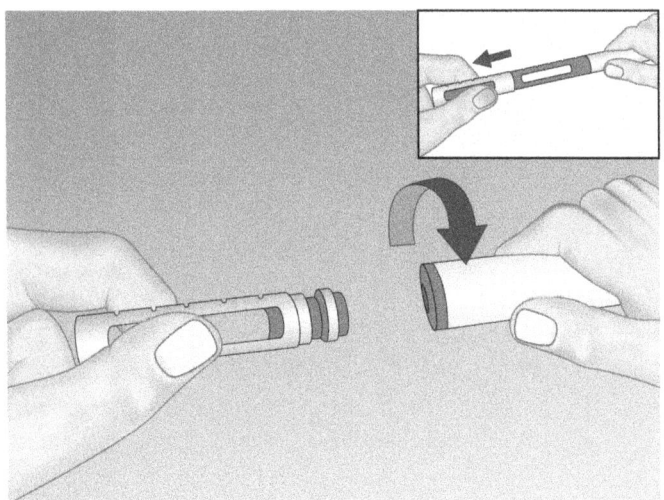

2. Press in the head of piston rod as far as it goes.

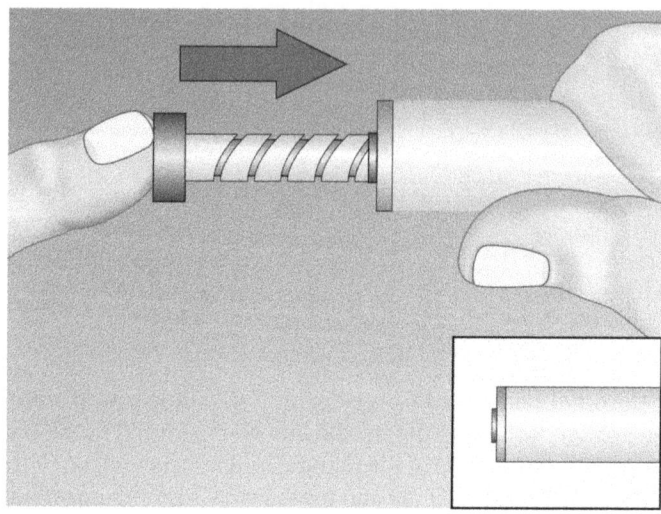

3. Insert insulin cartridge into the cartridge holder. Color-coded cap end goes in first.

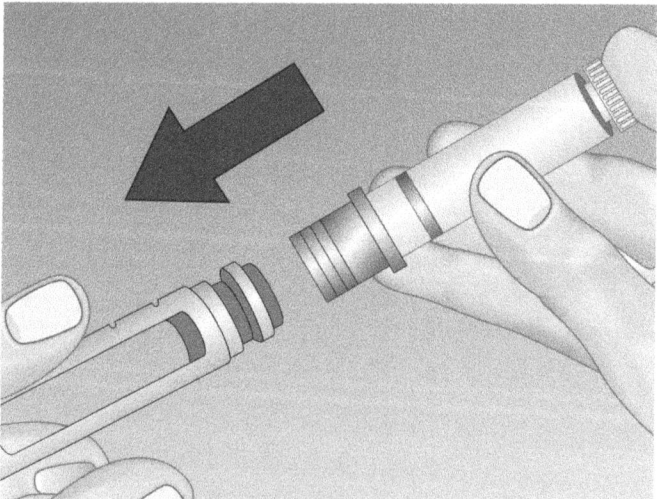

CHAPTER 9: Insulin Delivery Systems

4. Screw together the two parts of insulin pen tightly till the click is heard. Subsequently, screw on insulin needle.

   Note: Before inserting cartridge of cloudy insulin (e.g., Mixtard and Novomix), role it between the palms for about 20 times.

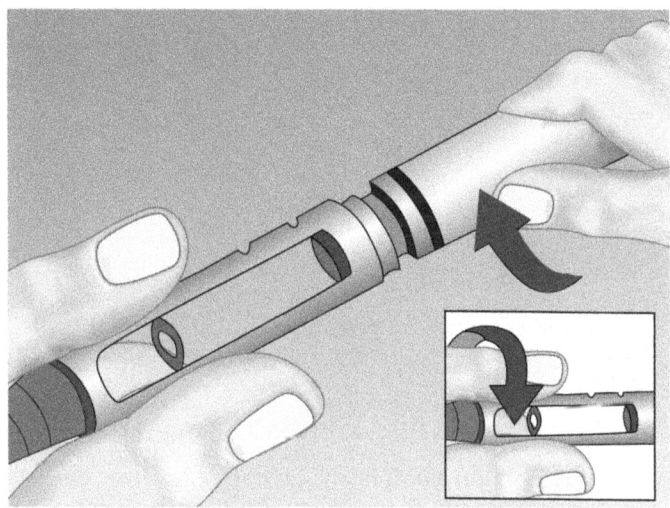

5. Prime the pen by pulling out dose button and turning it in clockwise manner to select 4 (4 units) in case of new cartridge.
6. Or, 1 (1 unit) in case of cartridge already in use.

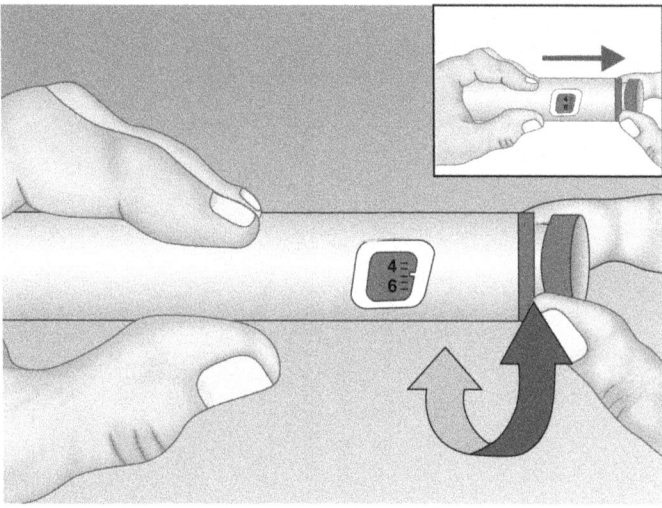

7. Hold the pen with needle facing upward and tap the cartridge holder to raise air bubble if any to the top of the cartridge.

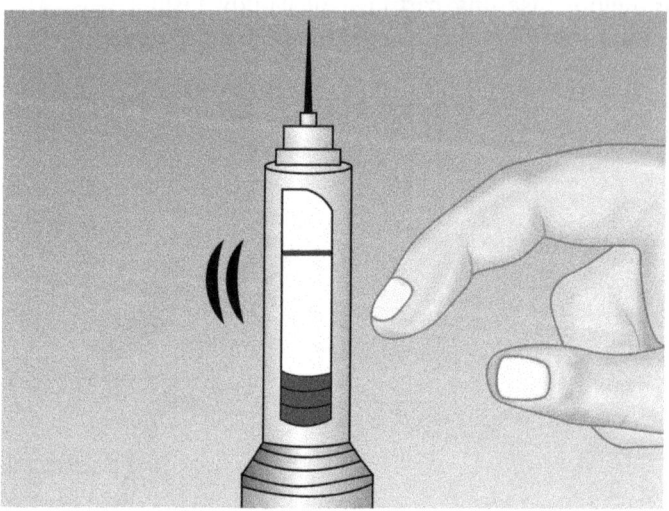

8. Press the dose button completely in until the dose display window shows 0. Confirm that a drop of insulin has appeared at the tip of the needle. This confirms that the pen is now primed successfully and is ready for use. If a drop of insulin dose does not appear at the needle tip, repeat steps number 5-7 till a drop of insulin appears at the tip of needle. Now, the pen is ready for use.

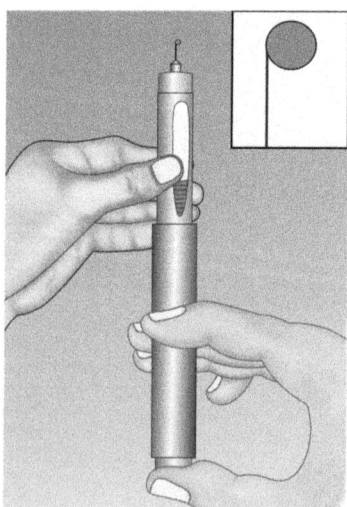

9. *Selecting the dose:* Pull out the dose button and rotate it clockwise till the required dose.

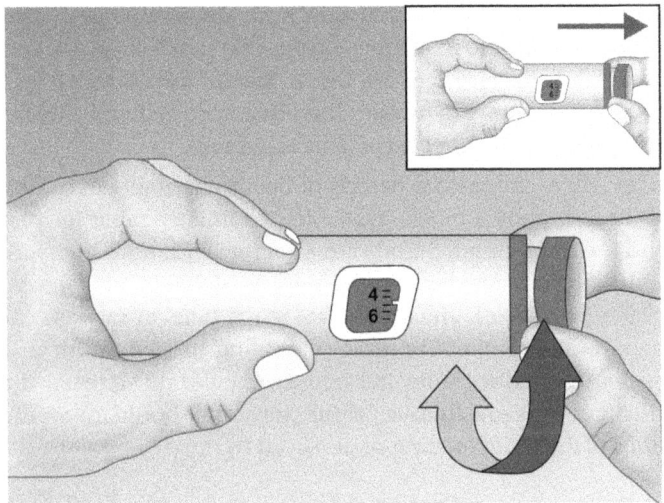

10. *Making the injection:* The actual injecting procedure and the sites of injection are the same for insulin injections through pen and syringes. To inject insulin through pen, press the dose button completely till the display shows 0 and you hear or feel a click. Subsequently, leave the needle under the skin for about 10 seconds. Then, withdraw the needle and replace the needle cap, followed by the pen cap. Please note that as per insulin manufacturer recommendations, the needle needs to be changed after each injection; however, those who need to economize, are using the same needle up to 3-4 times with proper hygienic care.

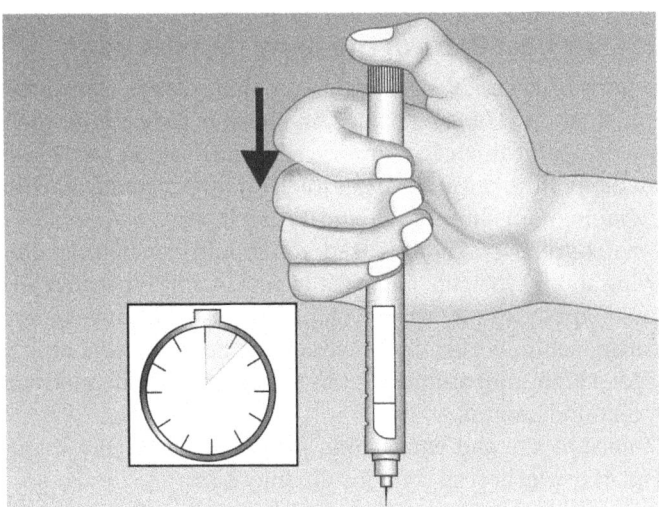

The procedure for injecting insulin from disposable pen is essentially same as that for reusable pen. Since disposable pen is available in ready-to-use form with insulin cartridge inserted at the manufacturer's level, first four steps described above are bypassed. This advantage of disposable insulin pen has to be traded with higher cost of insulin per unit.

Note: Today, there are several brands of insulin available in Indian market. Many of these brands are also available in forms suitable for pen devices along with the pens. Some brands are available with both the types of pens (disposable and reusable), while others are available in only one type of pen (disposable or reusable). Thus, there are many pens in market; each brand has its own branded pen. The exact operating procedure for a particular brand of pen may differ from the one described above, even though the basic principles are same. In case of difficulty, one should follow the specific instructions of the manufacturer of pen used by the patient.

Tips for Painless Insulin Injection

- Remove insulin vial/pen from refrigerator a few minutes before injection so that at the time of injection, temperature of insulin is more or less same as the room temperature.
- Wait for a minute after applying spirit or alcohol. Let alcohol evaporate before injecting.
- Use No. 32 needle for injecting insulin. Better still, use insulin pens for injecting insulin.
- Advance the syringe or pen in swift, linear manner, do not change the direction.

What are the Best Parts of the Body for Injection?

The best parts of the body for injection are those where a loose fold of flesh can be pinched up **(Fig. 4)**. Absorption speed is fastest from the abdomen and slowest from the thigh and buttock, while absorption speed from the arm is intermediate. Thus, one may prefer thigh for intermediate- and long-acting insulin, abdomen for short- and rapid-acting insulin, and arm for premixed insulin. Whichever part of body is used, you should vary the injection site each day, moving about 1 inch up or down and across. This is because an unsightly lump due to lipodystrophy will develop if you use the same spot repeatedly and because insulin is absorbed more slowly and unpredictably from such an area. After shift from animal insulin to human insulin, lipodystrophy has become very uncommon.

The injection site and your hands should be clean. The shaded circled areas **(Fig. 4)** depict best sites for insulin injection.

CHAPTER 9: Insulin Delivery Systems

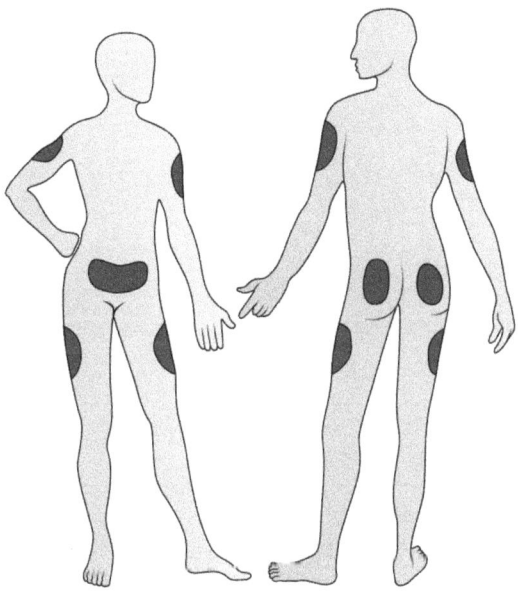

FIG. 4: Sites for insulin injection.

■ SUMMARY

In parallel, with the continuous improvements in the purity and the quality of insulin, there has been similar evolutionary improvement in the the systems used to deliver insulin. The currently used short and fine bored disposable needles for syringes and pens are poles apart as compared to blunt reusable metal needles and glass syringes. Pens have significantly improved accuracy and ease of insulin delivery. The pumps used for continuous sub subcutaneous delivery of insulin have become extremely high tech and have the capabilities of delivering insulin in an automatic manner due to the presence of sensors for continuous monitoring of interstitial fluid glucose and algorithms to analyse the data generated by the sensors and automatically adjust the insulin dosage.

In spite of all the developments, awful blunders occasionally occur due to mismatch between insulin syringes and insulin concentration in vials and due to faulty improvisation as regards insulin pens leading to metabolic derangement. Thus, it is a primary clinician's duty to continuously keep himself abreast with the latest developments in technology and develop hands on-experience as regards the available technology.

CHAPTER 10

Insulin Preparations Available in India

■ INTRODUCTION

The availability of brands and formulations of various insulin preparations is ever increasing. In the last few months, several companies have entered or reentered insulin market. Not only we have a choice of multiple branded generic human insulin preparations to choose from, but even the biosimilar versions of costlier insulin analogs are now available at significantly reduced cost. Furthermore, glargine, the most commonly prescribed insulin analog, has recently come under price control, and the competition from the biosimilar versions has further reduced its cost. All these happenings are a boon to our patients and it is hoped that more patients will be able to initiate and uptitrate insulin therapy in timely manner.

From practical point of view, besides having in-depth knowledge about pharmacokinetic properties, such as onset of action, peak time of action, and duration of action, the prescribing doctor should also have correct information about the availability of insulin in different formats (U/40 and U/100 vials, disposable/reusable pens, concentration of insulin in pens such as U/100 or U/200), retail price, brand names of formulations, etc. The author has made efforts to compile all the abovementioned data in tabular form and tried to keep it up to date. The practitioner can use the data as a ready reckoner and confidently write a technically correct and detailed insulin prescription.

■ INSULIN STORAGE

Unopened vials, cartridges, and pens should be stored between 3 and 8°C. The door or the areas outside the freezer compartment of the refrigerator should be used to store insulin. It should never be stored in a freezer compartment.

Opened vials and cartridges should be stored between 3 and 30°C. On the date of expiry, insulin should be discarded. Open vials and pens should be discarded 1 month after opening them. If stored outside the refrigerated enclosure, insulin vials and pens should not be exposed to direct sunlight or heat producing source. Those not having access to the refrigerator can store insulin preparations in current use in the coolest room of their house. In summer months, they can store insulin preparations in an earthen pot covered with wet cloth. While traveling in an automobile, do not keep insulin preparations in the luggage compartment or in a glove box under the dashboard. Keep them in an insulated pouch or around a slab of dry ice in a pouch. The dry ice should be kept in the freezer compartment of a refrigerator for about 8 hours and transferred to the pouch just before the beginning of travel. While breaking the journey, insulin-containing pouch should be carried along and never kept in a parked car with rolled up windows as the temperature inside the car rises significantly and reduces the potency of insulin in such a situation.

CONVENTIONAL HUMAN INSULIN

Table 1 shows all the conventional (Human) insulin available in India.

Table 1: Conventional human insulin.

Type	Insulin	Brands	Company	Available SKUs and their MRPs	Disposable device	Reusable device
Regular or short-acting insulin	• Human insulin • Regular	Xsulin R	Eris	Vial 10 mL (INR 157 and INR 310-U/100)	Eris 1 Pen (INR 560)	Xsulin Pen
		Actrapid	Novo Nordisk	Vial 10 mL (INR 390)	Flexpen (INR 569)	Novopen 4 (INR 1,499)
		Huminsulin-R	Lupin	Vial 10 mL (INR 174 and INR 539-U/100)		Humapen Ergo 2 (INR 1,040)
		Lupisulin-R	Lupin	Vial 10 mL (INR 178)		Lupisulin Pen (INR 1,049)
		Insugen-R	Biocon	Vial 10 mL (INR 178 and INR 518-U/100)		Insupen Pro (INR 1,299)
		Wosulin-R	Wockhardt	Vial 5/10/15 mL (INR 240-U/100, INR 178 and INR 196)		Royal Device
		Insuman R	Sanofi	Vial 10 mL (INR 147)		
				Cartridge 3 mL (INR 367)		Allstar (INR 977)
		Equisulin R	Koye Pharma	Vial 10 mL (INR 169)		Equisulin Pen (INR 1,200)
		Recosulin-R	Shreya	Vial 10 mL (INR 147)		

Continued

CHAPTER 10: Insulin Preparations Available in India

Continued

Type	Insulin	Brands	Company	Available SKUs and their MRPs	Disposable device	Reusable device
Intermediate-acting insulin OR NPH (neutral protamine Hagedorn) insulins	Human insulin Isophane	Xsulin N	Eris	Vial 10 mL (INR 157)		
		Insulatard	Novo Nordisk	Vial 10 mL (INR 149)	Cartridge 3 mL (INR 390)	Flexpen (INR 569)	Novopen 4 (INR 1,499)
		Huminsulin-N	Lupin	Vial 10 mL (INR 174 and INR 539-U/100)	Cartridge 3 mL (INR 427)		Humapen Ergo 2 (INR 1,040)
		Lupisulin-N	Lupin	Vial 10 mL (INR 178)	Cartridge 3 mL (INR 320)		Lupisulin Pen (INR 1,049)
		Insugen-N	Biocon	Vial 10 mL (INR 178 and INR 518-U/100)	Cartridge 3 mL (INR 214)		Insupen Pro (INR 1,299)
		Wosulin-N	Wockhardt	Vial 5/10 mL (INR 135 and INR 178)	Cartridge 3 mL (INR 213)		Royal Device
		Recosulin-N	Shreya	Vial 10 mL (INR 140 and INR 334-U/100)			
		Insuman Basal	Sanofi	Vial 10 mL (INR 140)			

Continued

Continued

Type	Insulin	Brands	Company	Available SKUs and their MRPs		Disposable device	Reusable device
Regular or short-acting insulin + Intermediate-acting/NPH insulin	Human insulin Premix 30/70 (Regular-acting insulin 30% + Intermediate-acting 70% insulin)	Human Mixtard 30/70	Novo Nordisk	Vial 10 mL (INR 178 and INR 496-U/100)	Cartridge 3 mL (INR 385)	Flexpen (INR 569)	Novopen 4 (1,499)
		Huminsulin 30/70	Lupin	Vial 10 mL (INR 174 and INR 539-U/100)	Cartridge 3 mL (INR 469)		Humapen Ergo 2 (INR 1,040)
		Lupisulin-M 30/70	Lupin	Vial 10 mL (INR 178)	Cartridge 3 mL (INR 385)		Lupisulin Pen (INR 1,049)
		Insugen 30/70	Biocon	Vial 10 mL (INR 178)	Cartridge 3 mL (INR 284)		Insupen Pro (INR 1,299)
		Wosulin 30/70	Wockhardt	Vial 5/10 mL (INR 157 and 178)	Cartridge 3 mL (INR 318)		Royal Device
		Insuman 30/70	Sanofi	Vial 10 mL (INR 167)	Cartridge 3 mL (INR 367)		Allstar (INR 977)
		Xsulin 30/70	Eris	Vial 10 mL (INR 178)	Cartridge 3 mL (INR 341)		Xsulin Pen (INR 560)
		Equisulin-M 30/70	Koye Pharma	Vial 10 mL (INR 169)	Cartridge 3 mL (INR 266)		Equisulin Pen (INR 1,200)
		Recosulin-M 30/70	Shreya	Vial 10 mL (INR 143 and INR 366-U/100)			

Continued

CHAPTER 10: Insulin Preparations Available in India

Continued

Type	Insulin	Brands	Company	Available SKUs and their MRPs		Disposable device	Reusable device
Human insulin Premix 50/50 (Regular-acting insulin 50% + Intermediate-acting 50% insulin)	Human Mixtard 50/50	Novo Nordisk	Vial 10 mL (INR 265)	Cartridge 3 mL (INR 385)	Flexpen (INR 569)	Novopen 4 (INR 1,499)
		Huminsulin 50/50	Lupin	Vial 10 mL (INR 174 and INR 539-U/100)	Cartridge 3 mL (INR 383)		Humapen Ergo 2 (INR 1,040)
		Lupisulin-M 50/50	Lupin	Vial 10 mL (INR 178)	Cartridge 3 mL (INR 368)		Lupisulin Pen (INR 1,049)
		Insugen 50/50	Biocon	Vial 10 mL (INR 220)	Cartridge 3 mL (INR 258)		Insupen Pro (INR 1,299)
		Wosulin 50/50	Wockhardt	Vial 5/10 mL (INR 157 and 230)	Cartridge 3 mL (INR 273)		Royal Device
		Insuman 50/50	Sanofi	Vial 10 mL (INR 167)	Cartridge 3 mL (INR 367)		Allstar (INR 977)
		Xsulin 50/50	Eris	Vial 10 mL (INR 133)	Cartridge 3 mL (INR 341)		Xsulin Pen
		Equisulin-M 50/50	Koye Pharma	Vial 10 mL (INR 169)	Cartridge 3 mL (INR 266)		Equisulin Pen (INR 1,200)
		Recosulin-M 50/50	Shreya	Vial 10 mL (INR 180 and INR 334-U/100)			

ANALOG INSULINS

Table 2 shows all the analog insulins available in India.

Table 2: Analog insulins.

Type	Insulin	Brands	Company	SKUs available		Disposable device	Reusable devices
Rapid-acting insulin analogs	Insulin aspart	Novorapid	Novo Nordisk	Vial 10 mL (INR 2,321)	Cartridge 3 mL (INR 851)	Flexpen (INR 1,052)	Novopen 4 (INR 1,499)
	Insulin aspart	InsuQuick	USV	Vial 10 mL (INR 2,321)	Cartridge 3 mL (INR 700)	InsuQuick VD Pen (INR 915)	USV Pen
	Insulin glulisine	Apidra	Sanofi	Vial 10 mL (INR 1,534)	Cartridge 3 mL (INR 761)	Solostar (INR 968)	Allstar (INR 977)
	Insulin lispro	Humalog	Cipla		Cartridge 3 mL (INR 990)	• Kwikpen (INR 1,131) • Kwikpen 200 IU/mL (INR 1,859) • Kwikpen Junior (INR 1,029)	Humapen Ergo 2 (INR 1,040)
	Insulin lispro	Eglucent	Lupin		Cartridge 3 mL (INR 990)	Kwikpen (INR 1,244)	Humapen Ergo 2 (INR 1,040)
Ultra-rapid-acting analogs	Insulin aspart	Fiasp	Novo Nordisk	Vial 10 mL (INR 2,021)	Cartridge 3 mL (INR 740)	Flextouch (INR 914)	Novopen 4 (INR 1,499)
Premix insulin analogs	Insulin aspart (30%) + Insulin aspart protamine (70%)	Novomix 30/70	Novo Nordisk		Cartridge 3 mL (INR 851)	Flexpen (INR 1,052)	Novopen 4 (INR 1,499)
	Insulin aspart (50%) + Insulin aspart protamine (50%)	Novomix 50/50			Cartridge 3 mL (INR 883)	Flexpen (INR 1,089)	Novopen 4 (INR 1,499)

Continued

CHAPTER 10: Insulin Preparations Available in India

Continued

Type	Insulin	Brands	Company	SKUs available	Disposable device	Reusable devices
	Insulin lispro (25%) + Insulin lispro protamine (75%)	• Humalog-Mix 25/75 • Eglucent Mix 25/75	• Cipla • Lupin	Cartridge 3 mL (INR 990)	• Kwikpen (INR 1,131) • Eglucent Mix 25 Kwikpen (INR 1,244)	Humapen Ergo 2 (INR 1,040)
	Insulin lispro (50%) + Insulin lispro protamine (50%)	• Humalog-Mix 50/50 • Eglucent Mix 50/50	• Cipla • Lupin	Cartridge 3 mL (INR 990)	• Kwikpen (INR 1,131) • Eglucent Mix 50 Kwikpen (INR 1,244)	Humapen Ergo 2 (INR 1,040)
Insulin co-formulation	Insulin degludec 70%/Insulin aspart 30%	Ryzodeg	Novo Nordisk	Cartridge 3 mL (INR 1,238)	Flextouch (INR 1,595)	Novopen 4 (INR 1,499)
Ultra-long-acting insulin analogs	Insulin degludec recombinant (100 IU)	Tresiba	Novo Nordisk	Cartridge 3 mL (INR 1,440)	Flextouch (INR 1,942)	Novopen 4 (INR 1,499)
Long-acting insulin analogs	Insulin glargine recombinant (100 IU)	Lantus	Sanofi	Vial 10 mL (INR 2,136)	Solostar (INR 769)	Allstar (INR 977)
		Basalog	Biocon	Vial 3/5/10 mL (INR 564/INR 822/INR 1,782)	Basalog One (INR 699)	Insupen Pro (INR 1,299)
		Basaglar	Cipla	Cartridge 3 mL (INR 731)	Kwikpen (INR 769)	Humapen Ergo 2 (INR 1,040)
		Glaritus	Wockhardt	Vial 10 mL (INR 2,101)	Dispo Pen (INR 769)	Pen Royale (INR 450)

Continued

Continued

Type	Insulin	Brands	Company	SKUs available	Disposable device	Reusable devices
		Basugine	Lupin	Vial 10 mL (INR 2,465)		Basugine Pen (INR 1,049)
				Cartridge 3 mL (INR 594)		
		Xglar	Eris	Vial 5 mL (INR 782)	Xglar One (INR 769)	Xglar Pen (INR 1,299)
				Cartridge 3 mL (INR 610)		
		Nobeglar	Mankind	Vial 5 mL (INR 822)	Nobeglar Uno (INR 749)	Comfy Pen (INR 1,299)
				Cartridge 3 mL (INR 610)		
	Insulin glargine recombinant (300 IU)	Toujeo	Sanofi	Cartridge 1.5 mL (300 IU/mL) (INR 1,400)	Solostar (INR 769)	Allstar (INR 977)
	Insulin detemir recombinant (100 IU)	Levemir	Novo Nordisk		Flexpen (INR 1,449)	

Note: The availability and retail price of insulin products can change from time to time. (SKUs stock keeping units)

CHAPTER 10: Insulin Preparations Available in India

SUMMARY

Insulin preparations are marketed in our country by many companies, each under their own brand names. Also, each company markets several variants of insulin having different pharmacokinetic properties, structure, concentration; and pack size. Vital logistic information as regards availability of various insulin preparations in various SKU's, their brand names, cost, storage and transportation requirements, etc., is given in this chapter to facilitate the process of prescription of appropriate insulin formulation as per the individual patient's needs.

Index

Page numbers followed by *f* refer to figure, *fc* refer to flowchart, and *t* refer to table.

A

Addison's disease 74
Adenosine
  diphosphate 21
  triphosphate 21
    generation of 20
Alanine 10
Alpha-glucosidase inhibitors 3, 49
Alpha-ketoglutarate 21
Ambulatory, goals for 37*t*
American Association of Clinical Endocrinologists 37
American Diabetes Association 37
Amino acid 44
  arginine 40
  removal of 44
  sequence of 38
    insulin 13
  structure 41
Antidiabetic drugs 41, 56, 89
Antivomiting medications 66
Anxiety 75
Aspart 46
Atherosclerotic cardiovascular disorders 33

B

Banting's conviction 5
Basal-alone insulin therapy
  advantages of 54
  disadvantages of 55
Basal-bolus insulin therapy 50, 59, 60
  dosage calculation for 58
  dose adjustment in 59
  full-fledged 52
Basal-bolus therapy 53, 58, 62*f*, 63*f*, 63
  component of 41
Basal insulin analog, long-acting 44
Basal insulinization 45
Basalog 26
Basal-plus 2 prandial insulin regimen 58
Basal-plus insulin therapy 53
Beta-blockers 32
Beta-cell 1, 19
  dysfunction 22, 29
  functional capacity 24, 50
  in pancreas 38
Better-fasting blood glucose control 48
Biosimilar drugs 25
Biosimilar insulin 15, 25, 26, 27
  products 15
Blood glucose 9, 65, 69
  concentration 16
  control 42
  level, control 1
  levels 75
    premeal 59
  monitoring of 70
  prevalent 48
  values 90
Bovine 10, 10*t*

C

Carbohydrate 1
  containing food 75
Cardiac arrhythmias 70
Cardiovascular disease 2
Cartridges 104
Cataract extraction 70
Confidence, lack of 34
Coronary artery bypass grafting 37, 70
Corticosteroids 32
Cortisol 75
Critically ill, management of 64
Crystalline insulin 38
Cyblex 26

D

Dawn phenomenon 53
Degludec 37, 44, 45, 46, 47
   U-200 14
Deintensification, opportunity for 58
Deoxyribonucleic acid, recombinant 11, 16
Detemir 37, 45, 46, 53
   insulin 44
Dexamethasone, use of 71
Diabetes control and complication trial 36
Diabetes mellitus 1
   insulin regimens in type 2 53
   management of 66, 67, 80f
   pathophysiology in 19
   temporary remission in type 1 50t
   type 1 1, 4, 12, 22, 27, 33, 41, 49, 51, 74, 82
   type 2 1, 12, 22, 23f, 24, 27, 30, 31, 36, 38, 41, 51, 67, 83
Diabetic ketoacidosis 56, 70
Diacylglycerol 21
Diamicron 26
Dihydroxyacetone phosphate 21
Dipeptidyl peptidase-4 inhibitors 27, 50
Diseases
   lifelong 36
   prevalence of 33
   progressive 33
Drowsiness 74
Drug regulatory authority 26

E

Electrolyte disturbances 70
Endocrine cells 1
Endocrinology practice, emergencies in 74
Epinephrine 75
Escherichia coli 11, 26
Euglycemic-hyperinsulinemic clamp study 31
European Medicines Agency 26

F

Fasting blood glucose 54, 56
   control 49
Fasting glucose, impaired 31
Fasting plasma
   glucose 32, 56
   insulin levels 32
Fat 1
   metabolism 22
Fiasp 37, 40
Fiasp niacinamide 14
Flying
   east (days shorter) 71
   west (days longer) 71
Free fatty acids 21
Freezer compartment 105

G

Genetic engineering technology 11
Gestational diabetes 66
Glargine 26, 37, 45, 46, 53, 62, 82, 300
   concentrated 44
   conventional 44
   short 43
Gliclazide 26
Glizid 26
Glomerular filtration rate 72
   estimated 2
Glucagon 10
Glucagon-like peptide-1 receptor agonist 2, 23, 27, 32, 50, 57
Glucokinase sensors 30
Glucose
   insulin-potassium infusion 69
   monitoring, component of 54
   regulation 29
   responsive insulin 16
   tolerance, impaired 31
   transporter 2 21
Glucotoxicity, effects of 58
Glulisine 39, 46
Glutamic acid decarboxylase 51
Glycated hemoglobin 16, 37, 57
   levels 79f
Glycemic
   control 55, 80f
   goals 36
      stringent 67
   management, principles of 67
   target 37, 64
   threshold 75
Glycogenolysis 30

Grip syringe 95
Growth hormone 75

H

Homeostatic model assessment 32
Honeymoon period 51
Hormonal response 75*t*
Hormones 25
Human insulin 10*t*, 14*f*
  conventional 106
  preparations, multiple branded
    generic 104
  structure of 20*f*
Huminsulin 86
  injection 89
Hydrochlorothiazide 32
Hyperglycemia 23*f*
Hyperglycemia 76
  correction of 1
  rebound 76
  severe 58
  management of 1, 2, 24, 64, 66
Hyperosmolar nonketotic
  coma 56
  state 70
Hypertension 33
Hypoglycemia 23, 44, 70, 74, 75*t*, 80*t*, 80, 88
  after exercise 77
  associated autonomic failure 76
  diagnosis of 74
  early morning 60
  episodes of 42
  fear of 33
  impending 83
  management of 74, of 77
  occurrence of 74
  preventing 83
  range 88
  role in prevention/correction of 75
  severe 74, 75, 79
  symptoms of 76*t*
  treatment of severe 78
  unawareness 76
  with insulin therapy 74
Hypoglycemic
  coma 74
  episodes 37, 44

Hypotension 70
Hypothyroidism 74

I

Immunogenicity 11, 26
Immunoglobulins 25
Immunology 25
Immunomodulators 25
Immunosuppressants 25
Infections 70
Infectious diseases complications 3
Infusion fluid, selection of 69, 69*t*
Injecting insulin
  procedure for 102
  use insulin pens for 102
Insulin 15, 22, 24, 106-112
  adjustment of basal or long-acting 71
  administration in
    principles of 49
    special situations 64
  after breakfast and dinner 61*f*
  allergy 73
  analogs 12, 14*f*, 17, 110, 110*t*
    indications of rapid-acting 40
    rapid-acting 38
    structural formula of 39*f*
    structures of long-acting 43*f*
  availability of 104
  cartridge
    insert 98
    refilling 88
  coformulated 47
  concentrated 14, 103
  containing pouch 105
  conventional human 106*t*
  deficiency, progressive 27
  degludec 45*f*
  delivery systems 81
  detemir, structure of 43*f*
  development 16*fc*
  discovery of 4, 5
    Banting 8
    long-drawn-out saga of 7
  dose of 9, 54, 58
  exact copies of innovator 26
  glargine 42
    primary structure of 43*f*
  glulisine, primary structure of 39*f*

in hospitalized 64
in management of diabetes 36
in pens, component of 104
in type 2 diabetes mellitus 51
indications for premixed 47
induced hypoglycemia 32
infusion rate 65, 68*t*
inhaled 12
initiation 52, 56*fc*
injection 84
   fear of 33
   sites for 103*f*
   tips for painless 102
interchangeable 26
intermediate-acting 40, 59, 60*f*, 63
lifelong injection of 17
lispro, primary structure of 39*f*
long-acting 11, 16, 40, 42, 62, 63
method of administering
   intermediate-acting 54
mixing and injecting 91
molecule 10
morning's short-acting 59
need 49
oral 17
pens 81
   reusable 82*f*
   stepwise procedure for using
      reusable 97
   use 83
pharmacokinetics 46*t*
pharmacology 38
physiology 19
premixed 12, 46
preparations
   in India 104
   pros and cons of premixed 46
principal action of 1
producing gene 11
pumps 82
   conventional 83
   indications for 83
purity of 9
rapid-acting 61*f*, 67
regimen
   alternative 69
   basal-alone 54*t*, 58*t*
   intensifying 56, 63
release, nutrient-related 21*f*
resistance 29

and diabetes 30
bedside tips to tackle 32
etiology of 29
methods of estimation of 31
prevalence of 30
secretion
   beta-cells for 24*f*
   pathophysiology of 22
secretory β-cell defects 22
short-acting 38, 48, 59, 60*f*, 61*f*, 65, 67
storage 104
structure and function of 19
structure of 10
syringes 84, 91, 91*f*, 103
therapy 7
   evolution of 9
   intensification of 57*fc*
   stepwise intensification of 55
treatment
   initiation of 52
   intensification of 56*f*
type of 10
U-200 short-acting 14
ultrarapid-acting 37, 40
use 33
vials 81
   use 83
Intensive care unit 37
International Diabetes Federation 37, 55
Intracellular glucose transporter 2 20
Islets of Langerhans 5, 11, 19, 30
   to diabetes 5
Isoleucine 10

L

Leprechaunism 29
Lifestyle management 32
Lipotoxicity, effects of 58
Lispro 46
   insulin 39
   U-200 14
   ultrarapid-acting 40

M

Mass-market insulin 10
Mastering self-injection technique 34
Medical nutritional therapy 1

Medical profession 28
Meglitinides 50
Metabolic functions
Metformin 25, 49
Microvascular complications,
    progression of 36
Mixtard 86, 89
  drawn 88
  injection of 87
Molecular weight complex protein 25
Myocardial infarction 56, 70

N

Needle facing, hold pen with 100
Neoglucogenesis 30
Neurogenic 76
Neuroglycopenic 76
Neutral protamine hagedorn insulin 12,
    16, 41, 42, 40, 46, 60
Niacinamide 40
Nonalcoholic fatty liver disease 33
Norepinephrine 75
Normoglycemia, progression of 31f
Novel insulin molecules 16
Novo Nordisk's aspart insulin 13

O

Obesity 33
Open-loop system 83
Osmotic 58
Oxaloacetate 21

P

Palpitations 75
Pancreas 4
  artificial 83
Pancreatic extract 6
  purification of 9
Pancreatic poly peptides 10
Peripheral tissue 22
Pioglitazone 2, 49
Piston rod, head of 98
Plasma
  C-peptide 19
  glucose 31, 68
  insulin 31

Porcine 10, 10t
Postbreakfast blood glucose values 90
Postprandial
  blood glucose 40, 58
  values 57
  hypoglycemia 38
  plasma glucose 56
Potassium chloride concentration 69
Prandial insulin dose adjustment 58
Prebreakfast hyperglycemia 60
Pregnancy
  glycemic management 66
  treating diabetes in 67
Preinsulin era, important research
    milestones in 4
Premixed insulin, using twice-daily 72
Protein kinase C 21
Protein metabolism 1
Psychological insulin resistance 34, 35
  in clinician's mind 34
  management of 34
Pulsatile insulin secretion 21f

R

Rabson-Mendenhall syndrome 29
Random blood sugar 56
Rapid-acting insulin 59, 72, 81
    analogs 33
Refrigerator 105
  freezer compartment of 104
Renal
  impairment 72
  transplantation 71
Research Society for Study of Diabetes
    in India 55
Ryzodeg 47

S

Saccharomyces 11, 26
Self-injection, correct technique for 95
Septicemia 51
Sera 25
Sliding scale method 33
Sodium-glucose cotransporter-2
    inhibitors 27, 32, 49
Somatostatin 10
Standard cocktail 69

Statins 32
Steroids, moderate-to-high doses of 32
Subcutaneous patches 17
Sulfonylureas, coadministration of 50
Sweating 75
Syringe
    air bubbles in 94
    multipurpose 87

T

Thiazide 32
Threonine 10
Tongue, dry 66
Tremors 75
Tricarboxylic acid 21
Tuberculosis 51

V

Vaccines 25
Valine 10
Vasoactive intestinal polypeptides 10
Ventricular
    dysfunction, left 68
    failure, left 70
Virology 25
Vomiting 40, 64, 66, 72
    persistent 66

Z

Zinc 12, 40
    in insulin suspension 41

EU GSPR Authorised Reprsentative
Logos Europe, 9 rue Nicolas Poussin
1700, La Rochelle, France
Phone: +33 (0) 6 67 93 73 78
E-mail: contact@logoseurope.eu

www.ingramcontent.com/pod-product-compliance
Ingram Content Group UK Ltd.
Pitfield, Milton Keynes, MK11 3LW, UK
UKHW051138270226
468476UK00003B/23